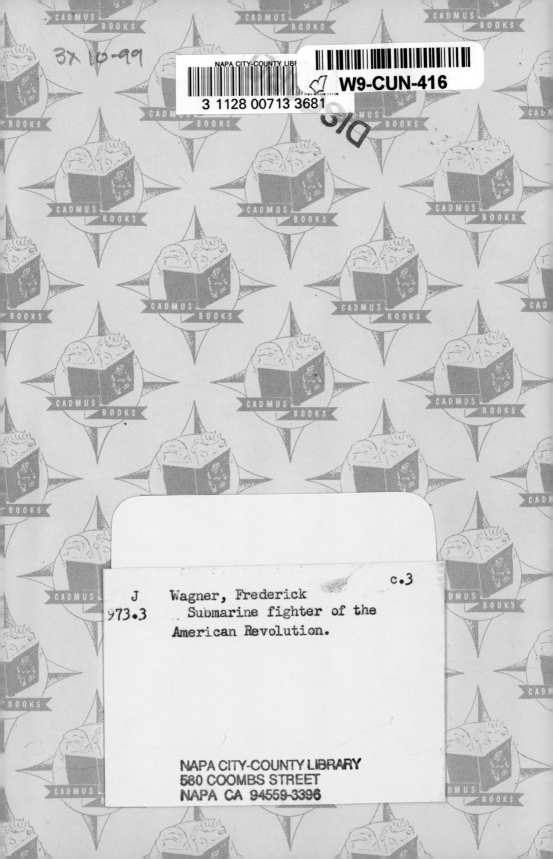

SUBMARINE FIGHTER
OF THE AMERICAN REVOLUTION

by

Frederick Wagner

The first machine built to travel underwater carrying explosives attacked the mightiest ship of the British fleet, Admiral Howe's Flagship, the *Eagle*, with Admiral Howe aboard, during the Revolutionary War. Built by a newly-graduated student of Yale University, David Bushnell had experimented with the *Turtle*, as his submarine was called, for a long time. No one had ever attempted to build such a craft for use in warfare, and David was the first to risk his life to prove that it could be done. During his first attempt, he was under the surface of water for 45 minutes. The compasses worked. He steered back and forth and came back up, triumphant. When the *Turtle* was tested against the Flagship, it was an error of judgment by the operator that caused it to fail, not the submarine itself. Next Bushnell developed underwater mines which touched off the Battle of the Kegs, after which he was captured by the British. Nathan Hale was his friend from Yale, and other famous people involved with the *Turtle* were Ben Franklin, Washington, Benedict Arnold and Aaron Burr. After the War, Bushnell mysteriously disappeared and the father of the submarine was silent about his great achievements and his important place in American history.

⚜

Classification and Dewey Decimal: American History (973.3)

About the Author:

FREDERICK WAGNER has co-authored many books with his wife, Barbara Brady. Mr. Wagner received his M.A. degree from Duke University then taught English at the University of Oklahoma and at Duke University. After serving in the army during the Korean conflict he came to New York City and has been promotion manager for a major book publisher.

Submarine Fighter of the American Revolution

THE STORY OF DAVID BUSHNELL

By Frederick Wagner

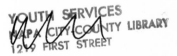
ILLUSTRATED

1966 FIRST CADMUS EDITION
THIS SPECIAL EDITION IS PUBLISHED BY ARRANGEMENT WITH
THE PUBLISHERS OF THE REGULAR EDITION
DODD, MEAD & COMPANY
BY
E. M. HALE AND COMPANY
EAU CLAIRE, WISCONSIN

For Barbara

Grateful acknowledgment is made for permission to use brief quotations from the following sources: *A Naval History of the American Revolution* by Gardner W. Allen, Copyright, 1913, by Gardner W. Allen, reprinted by permission of Houghton Mifflin Company; *Letters of Members of the Continental Congress*, Edited by Edmund C. Burnett, published 1921–1936 by the Carnegie Institution of Washington, reprinted by permission of the Carnegie Institution; *The Life and Works of Francis Hopkinson* by George Everett Hastings, Copyright 1926 by The University of Chicago, reprinted by permission of The University of Chicago Press; *The Papers of Thomas Jefferson*, Edited by Julian P. Boyd, © 1953 (Volume 8) and © 1955 (Volume 12) by the Princeton University Press, reprinted by permission of the Princeton University Press; a letter from David Bushnell to Henry Knox, dated January 2, 1783, in the collections of the Massachusetts Historical Society, reprinted by permission of the Massachusetts Historical Society; a letter from David Bushnell to Ezra Stiles, dated October 16, 1787, and a letter from David Bushnell to Thomas Jefferson, dated October, 1787, in the collections of the New Haven Colony Historical Society, reprinted by permission of the New Haven Colony Historical Society; and a letter from Benjamin Gale to Benjamin Franklin, dated August 7, 1775, in the Franklin Papers, Vol. 4, Part 1, No. 61, American Philosophical Society, reprinted by permission of the American Philosophical Society. The specific sources of these quotations are listed in the Notes at the back of this book.

Acknowledgments

FROM Massachusetts to Georgia many people—most of them librarians—went to great lengths to help in my search for material about David Bushnell. Without their great courtesy and kind assistance, usually far beyond the line of mere duty, this book never could have been written.

In Massachusetts I am indebted to Stephen T. Riley, Director, Massachusetts Historical Society. In Connecticut Mrs. Emery E. Bassett, Librarian, The Submarine Library, Groton, was not only most helpful in her replies by mail, but also gracious and informative on my visit to that unique library maintained by the Electric Boat Division of General Dynamics Corporation. At Yale University Library I owe a debt of gratitude to James T. Babb, University Librarian, and to both Jane W. Hill, Librarian, Yale Memorabilia Collection, and Dorothy Bridgwater, Assistant Head, Reference Department, who cheerfully helped in my race against deadlines. I also am indebted to Ralph W. Thomas, Curator and Librarian, New Haven Colony Historical Society; to Frances Davenport, Head, History & Genealogy Section, and to Doris Cook of the Connecticut State Library; to Elizabeth Knox of the New London County Historical Society; to Mrs. Frederic C. Hirons of Westbrook, and to the librarians of the Acton Library in Old Saybrook and the Westbrook Public Library.

In New York I wish to thank Robert W. Hill, Keeper of Manuscripts, The New York Public Library, and Arthur B.

Acknowledgments

Carlson, Curator of Maps and Prints, The New York Historical Society. A special word of thanks is due the staff of the Central Building of The New York Public Library—especially those in the American History and the Local History and Genealogy Rooms. In New Jersey Edith O. May, Reference Librarian, The New Jersey Historical Society; Lucien A. Le Jambre, Bordentown Historical Society; and the Curator of the Burlington County Historical Society all lent assistance. In Pennsylvania R. N. Williams, 2nd, Director, and Lois V. Given of The Historical Society of Pennsylvania kindly cooperated in the search for illustrations. Dr. Richard H. Shryock, Librarian, and Gertrude D. Hess, Assistant Librarian, American Philosophical Society, provided a copy of the letter from Benjamin Gale to Benjamin Franklin, which contains important new material about David Bushnell, and were extremely helpful in other matters. Mr. Irwin Richman, Assistant Historian, Pennsylvania Historical and Museum Commission, kindly furnished the item from Claypoole's *American Daily Advertiser*, which he found in his own research on Peale's Museum.

In Maryland I am grateful to Professor Vernon D. Tate, Librarian, and to I. W. Windsor, Reference Librarian, United States Naval Academy, Annapolis. In Washington, D.C., E. M. Eller, Rear Admiral, USN (Ret.), Director of Naval History, Department of the Navy, Office of the Chief of Naval Operations, provided help and information which I deeply appreciate. Victor Gondos, Jr., Chief, Army and Air Corps Branch, National Archives and Records Service, General Services Administration, furnished valuable material about David Bushnell's service with the Sappers and Miners. Daniel J. Reed, Acting Chief, Manuscript Division, The Library of Congress, also aided in my searches.

In Virginia I must, once again, express thanks to John L. Lochhead, Librarian, The Mariners Museum, Newport News. In Georgia Mary Givens Bryan, Director, Georgia Department of Archives and History, and Beatrice F. Lang, County Archivist, unearthed material about David Bush(nell), including a copy of his will, which I believe nearly everyone interested in the Georgia phase of Bushnell's life had long since given up hope of discovering; their amazing diligence has been a great help to me and has gone a long way toward clearing away the veil of mystery surrounding the last half of Bushnell's life. Information also was furnished kindly by Lilla M. Hawes, Director, Georgia Historical Society, and by Susan B. Tate, Library Assistant, Special Collections, The University Libraries, The University of Georgia.

And, moving west from the original United States, in Michigan Howard H. Peckham, Director, William L. Clements Library, The University of Michigan, was most courteous in supplying information and helpful suggestions.

I also am grateful to Merrick Jackson, Executive Editor, *Steelways*, published by American Iron and Steel Institute, and to Mary N. Plunkett, who kindly furnished the plates used on the jacket of this book of the painting by Anton Otto Fischer, which originally appeared in the January, 1951, issue of *Steelways*.

My editor, Joe Ann Daly, has once again provided unstinting encouragement and guidance.

FREDERICK WAGNER

Author's Note

"Who was David Bushnell?" a friend asked when he heard I was writing this book.

It was a fair question. David Bushnell had a passion for anonymity; he shunned publicity instead of courting it. He succeeded in avoiding fame, and today he has—unjustly—almost been forgotten.

"Who was David Bushnell?" He was one of the most ardent and least honored patriots in the American Revolution, a man who expended every shilling he possessed and risked his life countless times in the service of his country.

In an age that produced Benjamin Franklin and Thomas Jefferson, David Bushnell invented a machine so remarkable that Franklin himself received word from a friend that it was "not Equalled by any thing I ever heard of or Saw, Except Dr. Franklins Electrical Experiments."

This machine was not only the first American submarine, it was the first truly practical submarine in the history of all mankind, and the first submarine ever designed for offensive warfare. In addition, Bushnell devised and put into action the first mines ever used in underwater warfare.

This is the first full-length portrait of David Bushnell. It is not a fictionalized biography. Where gaps in the record exist, I have studied all the available evidence and made logical deductions, but I have not invented conversations, encounters, incidents or events. The facts themselves are remarkable enough.

No drawing of David Bushnell has ever come to light, and his friends and fellow soldiers did not leave any description of what he looked like. No doubt he was a plain man, plain in everything except what he did and the rare quality of his genius.

"Who was David Bushnell?" I hope this book explains who he was—and why we should remember him.

FREDERICK WAGNER

New York City

Contents

Illustrations

"Permit me to add a request to you to be so kind as to communicate to me what you can recollect of Bushnel's experiments in submarine navigation during the late war."

—THOMAS JEFFERSON to GEORGE WASHINGTON,
July 17, 1785

"Bushnell is a man of great mechanical powers, fertile in inventions and master of execution. . . . I then thought, and still think, that it was an effort of genius. . . ."

—GEORGE WASHINGTON to THOMAS JEFFERSON,
September 26, 1785

I ➤ "The Famous Water Machine from Connecticutt"

When the majestic frigate *Cerberus* sailed into Boston harbor on May 25, 1775, she had a prize cargo. On board were three British major generals—William Howe, Henry Clinton, and "Gentleman Johnny" Burgoyne. They had come to put down the little uprising led by a handful of colonists, the "rabble in arms" who had dared to oppose the policies of Parliament and the German king of England, George III.

Since April, shortly after the skirmishes at Lexington and Concord, His Majesty's troops in Boston had been besieged by this upstart group of rebels. "Gentleman Johnny," according to the rumor that ran swiftly through the British and American camps, was astounded at the situation.

"What!" he burst out scornfully. "Ten thousand peasants keep five thousand King's troops shut up! Well, let us get in, and we'll soon find some elbow room."

By October the only elbow room the King's troops had gained was on the mile-long Charlestown peninsula, which they won at the battles of Breed's Hill and Bunker Hill in June. Cooped up within Boston, His Majesty's soldiers found life more and more unpleasant as cold weather came on. Nerves grew taut, tempers flared.

1

The unruly, untrained Continental forces—some of them boys not yet in their teens—were equally miserable in their semicircle outside Boston. They huddled in Cambridge, and on the heights of Roxbury, and on Winter and Prospect Hills. Dysentery, fever and hunger swept through the ill-clothed, ill-equipped bands. And so did the bitter winter winds.

In a burst of patriotic fervor after Lexington, these men and boys had rushed off to Boston from Connecticut, New Hampshire, Rhode Island and other colonies, jubilantly answering the call to arms. They had been confident that hostilities would be brief, confident that their grievances against the Crown would be settled quickly. A number of them had enlisted for only five months. Now they were less confident. Each wretched new day they grew more aware that the insurrection—and the winter—were going to be long and grim.

In the countryside around Boston many of the townspeople and farmers had come to be almost hostile toward the undisciplined troops that passed through, day after day.

"When we advanced nearer to Boston," reported a private from Connecticut, "the inhabitants wherever we stopped seemed to have no better opinion of us than if we had been a banditti of rogues and thieves."

The soldiers continued to come, with their ox teams loaded with salt pork, dry peas, biscuits as hard as candlesticks, and, as the Connecticut private noted, "a barrel of rum to cheer our spirits and wash our feet, which began to be very sore by travelling."

Once at camp they found small comfort. Six soldiers were crowded into a tent about seven feet square. A blanket on the cold, damp ground served as a cot. The troops had one source of satisfaction: they had cut the British in Boston off from the rest of America.

Even this had a rub. As a port, Boston still was open to supplies from England. Worse, British cruisers operating out of Boston kept the New England coast from Portsmouth to New Haven in constant alarm. They were out in every direction. Parties landed to forage for fresh provisions. As they plundered they also burned and killed. Stonington, Connecticut, was cannonaded by the man-of-war *Rose.* In early October the little seaport of Falmouth (now Portland, Maine) was shelled from the sea and left a flaming ruin.

Even before this atrocity shocked the country, Massachusetts, Connecticut and Rhode Island had begun arming vessels to protect themselves and to cut the British supply lines. Eventually Congress authorized a Continental fleet. But this handful of vessels, valiant as it was, proved a sorry match for the celebrated Royal Navy.

When Molyneux Shuldham, Vice Admiral of the Blue and Commander-in-Chief of His Britannic Majesty's Ships in America, took command in October, the British fleet at Boston consisted of a 50-gun ship, seven frigates of 26 to 50 guns, eleven sloops of 4 to 24 guns, and five schooners of 8 to 14 guns. It was a small fleet even by the standards of 1775, yet large enough to strike awe and even terror into the hearts of the most daring American rebels.

Some of the shivering American soldiers who looked down on Boston and the mighty British fleet could smile in the midst of their misery. They had heard good news: a secret weapon was being built, and perhaps His Britannic Majesty's ships would prove not quite so invincible as they seemed. The weapon was a device that had been dreamed of for centuries, but never, until now, brought even close to realization.

From the camp at Roxbury twenty-seven-year-old Samuel Osgood (later the first Postmaster General of the United

3

States) wrote about it to his friend John Adams, then a delegate to the Second Continental Congress in Philadelphia.

"The famous Water Machine from Connecticutt is every Day expected in camp," Osgood scrawled. "It must unavoidably be a clumsy Business, as its Weight is about a Tun. I wish it might succeed, and the Ships be blown up beyond the Attraction of the Earth."

The "famous Water Machine"—a small submarine—was then being tested on the Connecticut River near Saybrook and out on Long Island Sound. She promised to be the world's first navigable submarine—and an offensive weapon as well.

Her inventor and builder—David Bushnell, Class of 1775 at Yale College in New Haven—knew the feat seemed impossible. He knew how many people scoffed at his attempt. But he was not a man to be stopped by impossibilities—or by scoffers. He had faced such obstacles before.

II ⤙ The Pochaug Farm ...
and Seeds of Rebellion

THE BUSHNELLS had been among the earliest settlers of the township of Saybrook in Connecticut. All were highly respected throughout the colony, but some had prospered, and some had not. Among the latter was Nehemiah Bushnell, David's father.

His farm lay about a mile northwest of the village green of Pochaug, known today as Westbrook. Pochaug was the west parish of Saybrook. The farm spread out over a hillside, which sloped down to the bank of the Pochaug River, so narrow it seemed little more than a stream.

The land on the farm was stony, but there were a few acres of good loam soil. Corn, rye, oats or hay could be grown when the weather was good and luck held. But Nehemiah Bushnell had not been born under a lucky star.

Although most men married before they were twenty, Nehemiah Bushnell remained a bachelor until he was twenty-nine. The farm yielded a meager living, barely enough to support himself, let alone a wife and children. And children usually were numerous, ten or more in a family, even though many perished in infancy.

After an uncommon streak of good fortune he felt in a

position to marry Sarah Ingham, a distant cousin. Their first child was born the following year, on August 30, 1740. They named him David.

Three years later Sarah was born, then Ezra in 1746, and Lydia four years after that. A dozen years passed before Sarah Ingham Bushnell gave birth to another child, a frail little girl named Dency.

It was a small family. With so few, each child had to bear a larger share of the work, and David, as the eldest, shouldered the largest burden. From early spring into late fall he worked, plowing the fields, sowing seeds, weeding and tilling the earth, harvesting the crops.

Every morning David was up early to get some chores out of the way before walking the mile or more to the schoolhouse, built the year of his birth, nestling at the foot of the hill west of the Congregational church.

School lasted from eight to five, and after school he had more chores to do out behind the steep-roofed farmhouse with its gray clapboards and central chimney. Water had to be drawn from the well or carried up from the river. Wood had to be chopped, berries picked and vegetables gathered. There were a few hogs to be fed, and at least one horse to be watered and groomed. The cattle frequently needed attention, and the barn always needed repairs.

One thing about David perplexed his father: he seemed to have little love for the land. True, he did more than his portion of the work, and he could be counted on to do it right. He was no slacker. But his heart was not in it, that was evident. Every moment he could snatch he was tinkering with gadgets. Bits of iron and wood and copper were always lying around the house and barn—just where Nehemiah would stumble upon them. The boy had more than an ordinary interest in mechanical things, and the amount of knowledge he

6

was storing up was astounding. But a farmer's son, thought Nehemiah, should put his best efforts into the land.

The boy was tireless. Even after dark he would not stop working. Sitting in the kitchen long after his brother and sisters and parents had climbed up the steep stairway to bed, he pored over whatever books he could lay his hands on. There was always the Bible to reread, or books borrowed from more prosperous neighbors. The flickering tallow candle provided a poor light, but from before sunrise until after sunset he had no time to sit with books.

Occasionally he let his attention stray from the page to dream of the future. The future he wanted lay about thirty miles away, at Yale College in New Haven. It might as well have been thirty thousand miles away, for all his chances of getting there. He was needed on the farm, and even if he could be spared, money could not. Sometimes he rode over to Saybrook Point to gaze at the original site of Yale. Nothing prevented him from dreaming—so long as he did not spend much time at it.

As David grew older, Nehemiah wondered more than once what he was up to. The boy kept to himself a good deal, working at his gadgets, studying his books. Some people were beginning to say that David was unfriendly, odd. But others—like John Devotion, the Congregational minister, or prosperous Elias Tully, or even Dr. Benjamin Gale, five miles away in Killingworth—remarked that the boy might possess a spark of genius. And Dr. Gale had a tongue like a whip: it could practically flay the skin from a man's back when he suspected humbug.

As for David himself, he paid little attention to what was being said. He was solitary, but not lonely. There was always Ezra to share his enthusiasms and marvel at his ingenious contraptions and amazing knowledge. The world around him was an exciting place.

A few miles to the south, where the Pochaug River emptied into Long Island Sound, Indians still had their wigwams. Although they appeared docile, David heard chilling stories of raids and massacres in the past, and from the western lands came new reports of ambush and murder as tribes fought back against the white invaders.

In cold weather wolves crept down from the hills to forage. Sometimes a panther appeared, and David or one of the other boys in the neighborhood, armed with a flintlock musket, would track him down to a thicket; the law allowed a bounty of £5 for his head. Marauding bears were always on the rampage, destroying great quantities of maize, tunneling under the barn door, battering their way into the milkhouse to lap up cream, wrecking havoc among the cattle and swine. Sometimes everyone in the village turned out to tree a mean one or drive him into the swamp. After he had been shot, the carcass was roasted whole, and the hunters had a feast.

But here was another thing about the boy that bothered Nehemiah. David was a crack shot; he knew more about guns than anyone else—man or boy—in the neighborhood. And yet, so far as Nehemiah could see, David did not really like to hunt any more than he liked to farm. It was the way the gun—and the gunpowder—worked that seemed to fascinate him.

And the sea and ships fascinated him, too.

Along the shore of Long Island Sound, bounding Saybrook to the south, were numerous small harbors. At Saybrook village itself, four miles east of Pochaug, was a splendid harbor in a cove near the mouth of the Connecticut River. Here coasting vessels often took shelter from bad weather. During the winter, when the river above was frozen over, the trading vessels back from foreign ports landed their exotic cargoes. David and the other boys liked nothing better than to watch these mysterious hampers being piled up on the docks.

Their interest had a practical side, too. If trade was good, there was a ready market for the products of their parents' farms. Coasting vessels carried grain, cheese, cider, flax and beef to Boston, New York, Philadelphia and the Carolinas. Flour, lumber and rum went to Gibraltar and the Barbary Coast, and flaxseed to Ireland. To the West Indies went ships laden with horses, cattle, sheep, hogs and lumber; they returned with molasses, cocoa, cotton and sugar.

For a while everything—even the Bushnell farm—seemed to thrive. The waters of the Sound abounded in salmon, bass and whitefish. Oysters brought a shilling a bushel, the price of one orange. There were shad held superior to any other in the country, so abundant that schools appeared in great waves coming through the water. They were salted and saved for food during the winter, or else shipped abroad in the trading ships.

As trade prospered, so did shipbuilding. It had commenced in Pochaug the year of David Bushnell's birth and was rapidly becoming a flourishing industry.

In the north parish of Saybrook was Uriah Hayden's shipyard, one of the finest in the colony. It was like a powerful magnet where David was concerned. He stopped by every time he could, and soon he was doing odd jobs here and there about the yard. The occasional shilling he brought home helped to reconcile Nehemiah to the boy's repeated absences from the farm.

During the years David was growing up, war or the threat of war was always in the background. It looked as though the world would never be at peace. At fifteen, he had a glimpse of what these savage struggles could do to human beings.

When the French and Indian War broke out between France and England, the British Governor of Nova Scotia feared, perhaps rightly, that the French Acadians in Nova Scotia might act as spies for France. He ordered them expelled. Driven from their farms and villages, their homes and barns burned to the ground, the exiles straggled down through the colonies. A band of them stopped not far from the Bushnell farm, at a spot to be known as French House Hill. Then they moved on; but their stories of scorched farms and flaming homesteads helped foster the dislike of the British that was taking root in the heart of the fifteen-year-old boy.

Seeds of rebellion were being sown elsewhere in the colonies. The ties with the mother country had been loosened over the years; now the rift widened between England and America. And when the French finally were driven from Canada, the colonies no longer felt themselves dependent upon England for protection.

Ill will grew as Parliament, oblivious to the temper of the American colonies, tried to close the western lands to settlement and restrict the profitable trade with the French West Indies. The Americans were developing a passion to manage their own affairs. Each new act of interference by a government far across the sea increased their rage.

The years passed, David grew older. Seventeen . . . nineteen . . . twenty-one. The dream of a college education seemed fated to remain only a dream. By day he worked, by night he read or planned devices that he would someday build.

Often, riding along the shore, he reined his horse to watch the ships, laden with cargo from the Connecticut farms and fisheries, sail past. And often, far off, he glimpsed the square-rigged ships of His Majesty's Navy. Were these ships—were any ships—really as invincible as everyone said? And did a ship always have to move along the surface of the sea? Startling ideas were stirring in his mind.

Then tragedy struck. At fifty-two, worn out by his struggle with the unyielding land, Nehemiah Bushnell died. Two years later Dency was dead.

It was often the custom for the eldest son to receive a college education as his patrimony, and for the next son to receive the farm. As David had never been able to get away to college, Nehemiah willed him the homestead, dwelling house and barn.

Although David and Ezra now plunged deeper into the work on the farm, they were—like their neighbors—caught up in the turmoil over the passage of the Stamp Act, the first direct tax Parliament had ever levied upon the Americans. All over Connecticut "the peoples Spirits took fire and burst forth into a blaze."

Throughout the colonies secret organizations sprang up to fan the fires of resistance. They called themselves the Sons of Liberty. During the summer of 1765 the Sons of Liberty promoted mass meetings, heated speeches, violent propaganda. When the Stamp Act went into effect on November 1, the church bells in the township of Saybrook tolled mournfully all day long, and ships along the shore flew their colors at half mast. In the village of Pochaug everyone—even children who had barely learned to speak—repeated the rallying cry, "Liberty, Property, and no Stamps."

The colonists who had accepted posts as stamp distributors, such as Jared Ingersoll in Connecticut, were special targets for abuse. At Lyme, just across the river from Saybrook, Ingersoll was accused at a mock trial (which he made sure not to attend) of having conspired with the Devil to murder his native land. His effigy was then whipped and hanged from a gallows fifty feet high. The scene was repeated in other towns and villages the length and breadth of the colony.

Finally the Sons of Liberty nabbed Ingersoll himself on the way from New Haven to Hartford, and in short order he resigned.

The story was the same in the other twelve colonies. Parliament at last gave way; the despised Stamp Act was repealed. But the damage had been done. As the crowds gathered to celebrate their victory around great bonfires, defiance of the Crown was strengthened.

On the Bushnell farm David and his brother labored tirelessly. As a team they worked well together, and between them was a strong bond. David led, and Ezra was eager to follow.

Then, in the summer of 1769, nineteen-year-old Lydia died. Mrs. Bushnell had long since learned to steel herself to adversity. She was strong and hearty, and life was a long way from being over (she lived to be more than a hundred). Two months after Lydia's funeral, she remarried. David and Ezra now were free to follow their own ambitions.

For David the choice was easy. As quickly as possible he arranged to sell his inheritance—the homestead, dwelling house and barn—to Ezra. After all these years the path to Yale had been cleared of all but two obstacles: he was twenty-nine, and he still had a great deal to learn before Yale would accept him.

College candidates usually were tutored by the local minister. The Reverend John Devotion, the Congregational minister, readily agreed to give David an intensive course of study. Although Devotion was testy and irritable, he was a good scholar and a perceptive man. Like David, he had an enthusiasm for perfection.

Then Elias Tully came forward with a helpful suggestion. Instead of riding on horseback to and from the farm each day, David could live in the Tully home in the heart of the village. There was a room available, and Mercy Tully set a bountiful table. David quickly accepted, and he plunged eagerly into two years of the hardest and most exciting work he had ever known. The boundaries of his world were expanding, and he meant to stretch them as far as he could.

III ➤ "A Bundle of Wild Fire
Not Easily Controlled"

EXCITEMENT CHARGED the air the year David Bushnell entered Yale. It was to rise to fever pitch before he graduated. "An hundred and fifty or an hundred and eighty Young Gentlemen," wrote one president of the college, "is a bundle of Wild Fire not easily controlled." And in 1771 the wildfire fed on the tinder of rebellion.

Conservatives in all the colonies were doing their best to bring about a peaceful reconciliation with England. Yet every time these men spread oil on the troubled waters, the Sons of Liberty struck a match to it. During a scuffle in the streets of Boston, five Americans were killed by British troops. Before the Sons of Liberty had finished reporting the event, it had been magnified into a deed of monumental infamy, to go down in history as the Boston Massacre.

More and more, the authority of the mother country was being questioned. The air was full of new ideas and new challenges, and the young men of Yale breathed deep.

As he jounced around in the stagecoach rumbling down the Post Road toward New Haven, David Bushnell had misgivings. His thirty-first birthday was a fortnight away, and by thirty-one most men had a wife, a family and a trade.

14

He had none of these. Instead, he was about to throw in his lot with a parcel of boys almost young enough to be his sons.

And he was poor, poorer than most. The pitiable sum due from the sale of the farm added up to his capital for life. Every shilling must be cherished, even hoarded; not a penny could be wasted. To the others, no doubt, his ways would seem odd and miserly.

His clothes, too, rough and poorly cut, were not the clothes of a gentleman. He knew there would be other farmers' sons at Yale, but would their shoes be so battered, their buckles so scratched, their white stockings so covered with darns? Most likely even his cocked hat, once so jaunty, would seem impossibly bedraggled. No matter. If he kept neat, clean and well-mended, even if it meant a patch upon a patch, he could not let shabbiness bother him. He knew there was nothing shabby about his mind.

Some things he would have to guard against. His temper, for one. It was hard to kindle, but slow to cool. And his impatience with slipshod ways, with anything less than perfection, that was something else to watch. There was no sense in stirring up a hornet's nest when he had so much to accomplish.

Meanwhile, the stagecoach passed milestone after milestone, carrying him nearer and nearer to the town of New Haven and his first glimpse of Yale. Like every loyal son of Connecticut, he knew its reputation. Only Harvard College in Cambridge and William and Mary in Virginia were older. Yale tended to be more conservative than Harvard— to turn out, as Harvard graduate John Adams noted, many a "pretty sensible, Yalensian, Connecticuttensian Preacher"— yet the rumor was afoot that it was fast becoming a nursery for Whig principles. And Whigs were radicals—at least in Tory eyes.

The coach dropped him near an imposing brick building, three stories high, higher by far than any building in the township of Saybrook. This was Connecticut Hall, he was told, and this was where he would room. The dormitory overlooked the town jail, and from time to time some of the students considered their lot not much better than that of the prisoners across the way.

In the next few days David investigated the other two buildings on the campus. The oldest building—narrow, wooden, and already somewhat rickety—was sky-colored College Hall, facing College Street and the beautiful town green beyond. It was used mainly as a recitation and dining hall. At meals the professors and tutors sat at a raised table, from which they looked down at the students, that "bundle of Wild Fire," and attempted to maintain order. The fare was plain, supper often just milk and a chunk of bread, or a hearty slice of apple pie. But these rations could always be supplemented at the buttery, where a few pennies would purchase sweets and cakes. Once a year at commencement, decorum was relaxed, the door was left unbarred, and the hall was used for dancing.

The small, almost square chapel, built of brick less than ten years before, with a steeple towering aloft, was the building David explored with the most delight. On the second floor were the library and the museum, and here he spent hour upon hour in the years that followed.

The museum was crowded with stuffed birds and animals, with fossils and stones. The college even possessed such marvelous contraptions as an air pump and a four-foot telescope. Although woefully inadequate by later standards, the apparatus was grander than anything David had dared hope to find.

The library boasted a handsome collection of books, gifts

from men such as George Berkeley, Isaac Newton, Richard Steele and Edmond Halley, many of whom had given Yale editions of their own works. At the first opportunity David pounced upon them avidly. There was an abridgement of the Royal Society's *Transactions*, where he could read about Halley's diving bell. Perhaps among Halley's writings he discovered some mention of an underwater mortar Halley had devised to blow up the decks of sunken ships and make salvage easier. If so, David could barely have suppressed a shout of triumph, for this supported a notion that had occurred to him. And at the first opportunity he planned to give it a practical test.

The tempo of campus life quickly caught him up, and his classmates became less a group of strangers. He was not so much out of place as he had expected. Of course, he was by far the oldest student, older even than some tutors. Yet even though the average freshman was sixteen or seventeen, the ages ranged from some in their mid-twenties to one boy just barely past eleven.

Freshmen were told their place and expected to keep it. "A Freshman shall not play with any members of an upper class without being asked, nor is he permitted to use any acts of familiarity with them, even in study time," ran one of the freshman laws. "Freshmen are obliged to perform all reasonable errands for any superior, always returning an account of the same to the person who sent them."

His thirty-one years gave David one advantage. Apparently he escaped having to run errands, a fate that made many a freshman's life hectic. It was clear from the start that David Bushnell would stand his ground, freshman laws or no freshman laws.

And from the outset some of the upperclassmen were his comrades. There was Abraham Baldwin, seventeen, the brilliant son of a blacksmith. A senior when David came to Yale, Baldwin remained a friend for life.

There were also two brothers, farm boys from Coventry, in the junior class. Both were good-natured, but Nathan Hale, the younger of the two, sixteen years old, was a popular favorite with professors and students alike. Erect, tall and vigorous, he was described by a classmate as being "as active as electric flame." Everyone believed he had a brilliant future in store, though he modestly held that his only ambition was to be a schoolmaster.

Like David Bushnell, most of the students at Yale had come to work hard (and those who had come to play had little opportunity). At six o'clock a rising bell summoned them to start the day, and anyone late to prayers was fined a penny. They labored over the Greek Testament and Cicero's orations; applied themselves to rhetoric, ethics and logic; figured away at arithmetic and geometry. Every week there were essays to write and lessons in divinity to be learned by heart.

The Professor of Divinity, Naphtali Daggett, was also president of the college. A big, lumbering man in his mid-forties, he had been the first to publish an attack in the press on Jared Ingersoll, the misguided stamp-master, and in a few years he was to take an even more courageous stand against the British, when they raided New Haven. Brave as he was, he was awkward as a speaker and downright inept as a disciplinarian.

Aside from several tutors—who were supposed to maintain order as well as teach—the Yale faculty consisted of only one other member, Nehemiah Strong, Professor of Mathematics and Natural Philosophy. Although unprepossessing, he was a kind man, and he had a keen mind. Evidently he regarded David Bushnell as an exceptionally promising student, for he allowed the freshman a special privilege: to conduct experiments without interference.

At last David had the equipment and the opportunity to try the tests he had thought about. The younger boys held him somewhat in awe, and he did little to encourage familiarity. As much as possible, he conducted his work in private. A true scientist, he preferred to perform his experiments without fanfare, cautiously, carefully, methodically. And he had no wish to alert the British to his tests: he did not want interference from authority. Gunpowder was an explosive subject in more ways than one.

David was convinced that he could make gunpowder explode underwater, and he succeeded. Although other men in the past—Edmond Halley, for one—may have achieved similar results, their methods were generally unknown. The method David used was conceived independently, from his own fertile imagination, not from someone else's work.

As always, there were Doubting Thomases. To prove his point, David assembled a group of influential gentlemen, sworn to secrecy, and put on a demonstration. Few details are on record. All that is known is that David placed two ounces of powder in a container, submerged it, and managed to get the fuse lighted. The underwater mine—the first one in history, so far as its observers knew—exploded, to the surprise of everyone except its inventor.

It began to appear that his discovery might soon have a very practical application. The Yale men, like the Sons of Liberty, were unwilling to let affairs revert to a state of complacency. There were many heated arguments in the rooms at night. A feeling of nationalism was growing, a spirit of self-sufficiency was abroad, and it was finding fertile soil in the minds and hearts of the men at Yale.

In September, 1772, when David's friend Abraham Baldwin graduated, commencement proved a good deal more lively than anyone had expected. At the ceremonies, it had been a

tradition for orations to be delivered in Latin. At this commencement, two of the Master's candidates delivered a dialogue in English, but it was the subject—"The Rights of
America and the Unconstitutional Measures of the British
Parliament"—that startled the audience.

"The Rights of America" . . . they were the subject of as
many fiery discussions among the Yale students as among the
Sons of Liberty, and to judge by David Bushnell's later activities, he participated ardently.

His stand was rewarded. In November, 1772, he was one
of the "four Sops which will make profitable members" (as
the minutes said) admitted into the Linonia Society. Despite
his solitary ways, David was making friends. Membership in
the Linonia was one of the most sought-after honors on the
campus. It was a secret student fraternity, founded "for the
promotion of Friendship and social intercourse and for the
advancement of literature," and Nathan Hale, now a senior,
was its moving force. Any underclassman he singled out for
approval felt that the future looked bright.

The Linonia even had its own library, and David is on
record as being one of the subscribers toward the purchase
of a copy of Rollin's *Ancient History*, one of the few luxuries
he allowed himself. Whatever money he could spare after
paying for bed, board and tuition went for his experiments.

Each year in April the Linonia celebrated its anniversary
with all-day festivities, starting in the morning with various
orations by the members. Then came the election of officers
for the following year, and sophomore David Bushnell found
himself one of five members elected to the Standing Committee. At noon the boys sat down to a rich banquet, and
after the banquet some of the members presented a play,
usually the latest success from London. What was left of the

afternoon was spent in "agreable Conversation & a Chearful Glass," and at five o'clock the group walked in procession across the campus.

All the while, David was working to increase the effectiveness of his mine. In the first trial he had used only two ounces of powder; for the second he decided to use two pounds!

This experiment required a more complex container. To the bottom of an ordinary hogshead he attached an oak plank two inches thick, then drilled a hole through the head and the plank. Into this hole a wooden pipe was inserted, leaving a few inches protruding beneath the plank and above the head. Over the lower end of the pipe he fitted a wooden bottle, and it was this bottle that contained the two pounds of powder. Once the pipe was filled with powder, it made an adequate fuse.

The next step was to load the hogshead with stones until it sank down in the water, leaving only an inch or so around the rim not submerged. Everything now was ready; witnesses were at hand to observe the results.

A match was put to the priming, and the onlookers fled, throwing themselves to the ground at a safe distance. Breathless, they watched the spot in the water where the hogshead bobbed up and down. Then, after a tense moment or two, the contraption blew up with a tremendous explosion, casting a great body of water along with stones and debris many feet in the air. No one could challenge the success of the demonstration.

In the months that followed, David made experiment after experiment, some of them with even more than two pounds of powder, and each of them produced a very violent explosion. The results, he later wrote, were "much more than sufficient for any purposes I had in mind."

The purposes he had in mind—like the steps being taken by some of the colonists—were drastic. They required a submarine mine or torpedo capable of blowing up the mightiest ship ever built. He had the plans all drawn when events outside the campus exploded nearly every hope of peace.

IV ➤ "Rise! Sons of Freedom!"

AT TIMES Parliament seemed deliberately bent on provoking the colonies. Take the Tea Act of 1773. Its provisions enabled the London owners of the East India Company to market tea in America at a cheaper price than colonial merchants—or even colonial smugglers—could afford to sell it.

The hot-blooded Bostonians, victims of so many indignities at the hands of the British, refused to sit back passively and suffer still another insult to their pride and their pockets. On a bright and frosty December night the cry went forth, "Boston Harbor a tea-pot tonight!" A mob of men—some dressed as Mohawk Indians, some with faces blacked, some without any attempt at disguise—rushed down to Griffin's Wharf and boarded three ships lying at anchor with cargoes of the East India Company's tea aboard. In little more than two hours, working feverishly in the cold sea breezes, the mob dumped all the tea, 342 chests full, into Boston Harbor.

News of this Boston Tea Party sped south like an arrow, striking a responsive chord throughout the colonies. Similar episodes, on a smaller scale and much less publicized, occurred elsewhere. Letters from home brought David news of what had happened in Lyme, across the Connecticut River from Saybrook. A peddler from Martha's Vineyard dared to come riding into town on horseback with a bag of East India

23

tea. The Sons of Liberty collared him and his tea, kindled a fire, and dumped the detested tea into the flames, where it burned to ashes. The peddler felt lucky to escape unsinged.

All throughout 1774 David struggled to perfect his submarine mine, or torpedo. What had started out as a daring experiment now promised to have tremendous potential for the patriot cause, if a rebellion actually erupted. A weapon such as this might well give the patriots the upper hand. He knew that it would require a powerful amount of powder, and he knew that the mechanism would have to run smoothly, with no margin for error.

Day after day, sitting in his small room in Connecticut Hall, David took quill pen in hand and bent over the paper tacked down on his drafting board. Slowly, carefully, he drew up his designs, making sure to test each step on a small-scale model. The final device would have to be gigantic, large enough to hold nearly 150 pounds of powder. This amount, he calculated, was needed to destroy one of the Royal Navy men-of-war, provided the course of events demanded such a drastic step.

The final design he settled upon was as simple as it was ingenious. The "powder magazine," as he called it, was to be shaped like an egg and made of two blocks of oak hollowed out and then fitted together, bound by iron bands. It was designed to be lighter than water, even when filled with powder, so that it would float up against the bottom of whatever ship to which it might be attached.

In addition to the powder, the magazine enclosed a firing device. This consisted of a clockwork mechanism, which could be set to run any length of time up to twelve hours. When it had run its course, it unpinioned a strong lock resembling a gunlock, provided with a good flint to insure against a misfire.

To prevent the clockwork mechanism from starting ahead

of time—or from being set off by accident—a long screw was provided, passing from the outside of the magazine to the inside, fixed so as to lock the movements of the clock. Once the screw was removed, the clock began ticking.

At last he achieved a design that worked to perfection in smaller models. There was no reason to believe it would not be equally efficient in the full-scale magazine.

Now all he had to do was create a vehicle to carry the torpedo underwater to its target.

He had it all figured out in his head, and he itched to be away from Yale, to be home at Saybrook where he could devote every moment to the building of it, free from curious eyes. In this case, tests with models would not do. The "submarine," as he called it, would have to be built to size.

During this time the political upheaval outside the campus continued to keep the students in ferment. In December some classes voted to give up drinking tea until import duties were taken off. It was a mild gesture of defiance, yet an omen of more violent demonstrations to come.

A few days later the college closed for three weeks, the first winter vacation in its history, and when classes resumed in mid-January of 1775, the country was on the verge of open rebellion. Everywhere, troops of militia were training intensively, and in February the students took steps of their own.

A company of recruits drawn from all the classes was organized. In long coats, knee breeches and cocked hats, the students marched snappily up and down the campus, drilling with weighty flintlock muskets. Soon the company was winning praise for its first-rate precision and discipline, and the boys never doubted their ability to defend Yale against the enemy if worst came to worst—as it seemed to be doing. The enemy, of course, would be the soldiers of King George III, actually still their lawful ruler.

Up in Boston, the simmering resentments boiled up into a seething revolt. On April 19 General Gage, the British commander in Boston, sent his troops to seize stores laid up by the provincial militia. The redcoats ran headlong into trouble. At Concord and Lexington the minute men, armed and on the defense, were waiting. By the time the British troops staggered back to Boston, everyone—Tory and Whig alike—knew that the fearful day had arrived. Civil war was inevitable.

About noon on Friday the twenty-first, news of the skirmish burst upon New Haven and the halls of Yale. "This filled the country with alarm," wrote one of the students in his diary that night, "and rendered it impossible for us to pursue our studies to any profit." With drums beating and rumors flying, "the bundle of Wild Fire" at Yale got completely out of hand, and the school term was brought to a close nearly two weeks before the usual date for vacation.

A bold sophomore, Nathaniel Chipman (who would one day become the chief justice of Vermont), wrote an ardent poem and dared to have it published over his name in the New Haven newspaper:

> Rise! sons of freedom! close the glorious fight,
> Stand for religion, for your country's right.
> Resist the tyrant, disappoint his hopes,
> Fear not his navies, or his veteran troops.

Chipman was well aware that such open defiance of the Crown could lead to the gibbet.

David Bushnell made no public proclamation of his hatred of the British. He had his own plans for disposing of the tyrant's navies, and the less the British knew about what he was doing, the better.

One of the townspeople who promptly answered the call to arms was the commander of the Governor's Guards in

New Haven, a dark-skinned, stocky man with jet-black hair. Once he had been an apothecary and a bookseller. Now he was a man of property, the proud owner of a splendid mansion, storehouses, wharves and vessels. He was fond of show, he was headstrong, and he was a man made for bold and desperate enterprise.

Immediately he called out his men and proposed starting for Lexington. About forty agreed to go. He then asked the town fathers to furnish his troops with ammunition. Their flat refusal sent him into a cold fury.

He bided his time overnight, but he was not a man to brook interference. As one of his soldiers later said, "He was our fighting general, and a bloody fellow he was. He didn't care for nothing; he'd ride right in."

The next morning the hot-headed patriot marched his troops to the house where the councilmen were in session, lined the company up in front, and sent in word that if the keys to the powder house were not handed over in five minutes, he would command his men to break in and help themselves. The threat was effective. The keys were handed over, the ammunition obtained, and soon the volunteers were on their way. Word went round that here was a hero of whom New Haven could be proud forever. As it turned out, they would never forget him. This intrepid patriot was Captain Benedict Arnold.

A good many of the Yale students set out for Cambridge, tagging along behind Arnold's troops, who were slick and smart in white breeches and scarlet coats faced and trimmed with buff. If David was among them, once he arrived at Cambridge he had his first real glimpse of the assembled might of the British Navy. He also witnessed incredible confusion among the milling throngs of colonial rebels.

Upwards of thirty thousand men had responded to the

news of Lexington, many of them dashing off direct from the fields where they had been plowing, without stopping to change their clothes. Some had come with their muskets, and some had come with only their bare hands for weapons. There was no discipline, no organization, little ammunition and not much food. Yet there was almost a holiday air among the crowds. Many of the men and boys at Cambridge still considered this war a lark. Few on either side dreamed that eight years of bitter conflict lay ahead.

If David actually went to Boston, he did not tarry long. With all the confusion, one body more or less made little difference. He had something more important to contribute. The plans for his "sub-marine" were all drawn up. The sooner he built her, he thought, the sooner the fight with England would be over. So he rushed back to Saybrook as hastily as others were rushing to the lines at Cambridge.

From the outside, the craft would look like the shells of two mammoth tortoises joined together, seven-and-a-half feet long and six feet high. The entry hatch at the top resembled a flat-crowned hat with a broad brim. In the crown, eight small windows—two in front and on each side, one in back and on the top—would provide light on the surface. The craft was designed to float with the primitive conning tower barely awash. The windows also allowed the one-man crew to see where he was going.

A valve in the keel would admit water to submerge; a forcing pump would eject it to ascend. For motive power there were to be three pair of oars, those in each set crossed like the arms of a windmill and fixed to the tip of an iron rod entering the interior of the vessel. One pair was for rowing forward or backward, one for turning right or left, and one for moving up or down. In principle they worked like a crude screw propeller. Finally, a rudder attached to a tiller within could be used for steering and for rowing forward as well.

Although men in the past had talked of building underwater vessels, no one had ever devised a machine like this. Two centuries before, William Bourne, an English innkeeper, had written of "a Ship or a Boate that may goe under the water unto the bottome," but the record does not indicate that he ever built her. In 1624 Cornelius van Drebbel had constructed a submersible boat that could submerge and ascend but that could not be navigated forward or backward. This boat was tested on the Thames, supposedly with King James I as a passenger. A brief mention of the boat and the test on the Thames had appeared in Thomas Birch's edition of Robert Boyle's *Works*, and a copy of this was in the Yale library at the time David was a student. From it, however, he could not have gleaned much practical information.

There had been others who had talked and dreamed of submarine boats, yet done nothing about them. Not until David Bushnell did anyone set out to build a fully practicable submarine vessel, and a submarine designed to go to war.

David knew what a staggering task he had undertaken, and he knew how expensive it would prove. Yet until he could demonstrate the capabilities of his submarine, there was small hope of financial help from the Governor of Connecticut, and even less chance of any aid from the Continental Congress. He had no choice: if the submarine was to be built, he would have to use his own money. And he meant to see the project through, if it took every shilling he possessed.

First of all, he needed a secluded spot for construction. Poverty Island, out in the Connecticut River, seemed a suitable site. Long since eroded away by the river, the island was then not far from Sill's Point, near the Saybrook ferry. It seemed unlikely that any British ships or British soldiers would come snooping around, but to prevent idle speculation he built a shed to conceal the work that would be going on. Then he gave out the story that he had become a fisherman and that the shed housed the reel on which he wound his seine.

The best way to keep a secret, he knew, was to keep it to himself, and he would have preferred to do all the work on the craft alone. But it was too big a project for one man to handle.

Fortunately, Ezra was eager to help. Although he had rushed off to enlist soon after the skirmishes at Lexington and Concord, military discipline was free and easy. Men went home to tend their farms almost whenever the whim moved them, and Ezra had no trouble in obtaining leave.

But Ezra's help still was not enough. David also needed an ironmonger. The entry hatch was to be brass, hinged to a broad elliptical iron band. Iron hoops were to go around the craft to strengthen it. Wherever the iron rods supporting the rudder and oars entered the vessel, David noted, "the joints were round, and formed by brass pipes which were driven into the wood of the vessel. The holes through the pipes were very exactly made, and the iron rods which passed through them were turned in a lathe to fit them."

Even with so few aware of his secret project, David still had to proceed cautiously and deviously. Even at Saybrook there were Tories—loyal to the British cause—and some of them kept quiet about their sympathies. That way they could learn more. David had no way of knowing which of his neighbors might be the one to betray him to the British. Gossip—even curiosity—could prove his downfall and possibly his death.

As construction started, he took every precaution to make the craft watertight and seaworthy. The seams between the oak timbers were corked and then tarred over. The joints were made so precisely that no water could seep in. The iron band to which the entry hatch was hinged also strengthened the wooden hull against the great pressure of water beneath the surface. Within, for the same purpose, strong beams buttressed the sides and doubled as a seat for the operator.

For a month he—and often Ezra, too—labored nearly round the clock. The craft was almost completed when a sobering fact brought David up short: classes were due to start again at Yale. The submarine was so close to realization he was tempted not to return. But the dream of a college education had once been as strong as his dream of a submarine now was. He could not toss away all those years of effort. It was risky to leave the submarine in the shed, but she was such a radical departure from all recognized boats that anyone stumbling upon her by accident would probably not be able to figure out what she was meant to be. When the day came to travel back to New Haven, David, his bags packed, was waiting for the stagecoach.

By the first of June, when classes actually began, most of the students had drifted back. Almost at once the campus was in an uproar. The hot-blooded young rebels discovered that at least one dissenter was in their midst: sophomore Abiathar Camp, Jr., of New Haven.

Groups gathered in Connecticut Hall and College Hall and before the chapel to discuss reports that Camp was "unfriendly to the just Liberties and Privileges of America." A committee of sophomores was appointed to examine the truth of the reports. Camp belligerently refused to cooperate. The committee then sent him a letter, demanding that he "either clear up your character, or let us certainly know that you are a profess'd enemy to your much injured country." Otherwise, they said, "We must take it for granted that those reports are real facts, and act upon them according to the best of our judgments."

31

Camp was not intimidated. He immediately dashed off an impudent reply in doggerel verse and dispatched it to his fellow sophomores:

> To the honorable and respectable Gentlemen
> of the Committee now residing in Yale College:
>
> May it please your honors, ham - ham - ham -
> Finis cumsistula popularum gig,
> A man without a head has no need of a wig.

His insolence was not calculated to soothe tempers. The sophomores referred the matter to a committee representing all the classes at Yale. This bold group declared openly that the student body was firmly behind the resolutions recently passed by the Second Continental Congress in Philadelphia, resolutions which put the colonies in a state of defense against the mother country. The allegiance of Yale to the American cause was now beyond question.

As for Abiathar Camp, the committee summed up the evidence against him as follows:

> That said Camp said he would by no means stand by the doings of Congress; that all those who recommended the doings of Congress, or justified the destroying of Tea at Boston, were a pack of d——d Rebels; and further, said Camp, if he was at home and the Liberty Party should rise against the Administration, he would fight on the ministerial side till he had kill'd a number of the Rebels (as he call'd them) before they should kill him; and further said, if he was advertised by the Committee, or neglected by College, he would only treat them with ridicule.

This was more than the Whig students could tolerate. After hearing the evidence the committee resolved unanimously to treat Camp as an enemy to his country and to sever all relations with him. A proclamation was nailed to the door of the dining hall, advertising him as a traitor. Camp escaped lightly; elsewhere, Tories were being decorated with tar and feathers.

Even though Camp flaunted his Tory sympathies, there were other Loyalists on the campus who kept their sentiments to themselves, watching for a chance to report rebel activities to the British authorities. These were the ones who presented such a danger to David. To protect himself he did not breathe a word about the submarine that lay, nearly completed, back at Saybrook.

Then, from north and south, exciting news converged upon Yale. From Massachusetts came word of the valiant American stand at Breed's Hill and Bunker Hill, where the provincials had inflicted appalling casualties upon a vastly superior British force. And from New York came word that General George Washington, on his way to assume command of the American troops at Cambridge, would be passing through New Haven.

On Wednesday, June 28, Washington rode into town, tall and erect in the saddle. At forty-three, he was a man to inspire confidence. His chin was firm, his mouth determined, and his wide-set blue-gray eyes were calm and steady. In his blue coat with buff-colored facings, a rich epaulette on each shoulder, and a black cockade on his hat, he cut a splendid and heroic figure.

Among those in his retinue Major General Charles Lee provided a vivid contrast. One year older than Washington, this volatile Welshman was rough in speech, sloppy in dress, moody, temperamental, and undeniably brilliant. He was one of the most colorful and controversial personalities the Revolution brought to prominence.

The students at Yale had been preparing for Washington's arrival. On Thursday morning the General accepted an invitation to watch them drill, and none of them ever forgot how warmly the Commander-in-Chief praised the demonstration. Afterwards the students and two companies of New Haven troops escorted Washington and his retinue out of town as far as Neck Bridge. Leading the students with fife or drum was a sixteen-year-old freshman, Noah Webster.

On July 25, when examinations were over, the college officials decided to pass out diplomas immediately, instead of waiting for the usual public commencement ceremonies in September. Of the thirty-five seniors, none could have been more eager to start off than David. He had important business elsewhere.

V ⊱ "You May Expect to See the Ships in Smoke"

THE YEARS at Yale had been hard, busy, eventful, and now they were over. Toward the end, ironically, David was so impatient to be gone that he gave little thought to what he had achieved. Despite sizable odds, he had come through with a degree. No longer was he simply a farmer of Saybrook: he was a graduate of Yale.

His thoughts were on the future. Even though British troops were bottled up in Boston, British ships still commanded the sea lanes, and the sooner he set about blowing them to pieces, the better.

Making all haste back to Poverty Island, David began putting the finishing touches to the submarine. Ezra was now a sergeant in the Third Company of the Seventh Connecticut Regiment; his lieutenant was David's friend from Yale, Nathan Hale, who had already abandoned school-teaching for soldiering. But, once again, Ezra was able to get home to help. They were a team, he and David, and he would come whenever needed.

With the frame at last finished, the fittings installed, and the hull properly caulked, the submarine was ready for an exhaustive and arduous series of tests. Nothing was to be left to chance. When the moment for attack came, David was determined that the submarine should not fail because of an oversight. The *Turtle* must accomplish her mission.

The *Turtle* . . . David had compared the craft to two shells of a tortoise, and the phrase was apt. When the finished vessel lay on the shore of Poverty Island, she looked exactly like a clumsy turtle. At first the name was used almost derisively, but soon it was used with affection—and pride.

From the very start, David realized that a skilled navigator was crucial to the success of his operation. Even though the machine functioned perfectly, human error could cause a fiasco. A man of exceptional strength was needed to steer the rudder and crank the propeller at the same time. He must be fearless, too, to venture underwater in this strange contraption, towing an armed mine. David was fearless enough, but he was already subject to spells of illness that hampered his efforts. Nevertheless, he made the first tests himself.

The momentous day arrived. Waiting until after dark, David and Ezra hoisted the *Turtle* aboard a sloop and sailed down the Connecticut River out into Long Island Sound.

David squeezed through the submarine's entry, which was barely large enough to admit his body. For safety, he had designed this entry hatch, or conning tower, so that it could be screwed down tight, or unscrewed, either by the operator within or by someone on the outside. Either way, if something went wrong, the one-man crew was assured of escape —provided the *Turtle* was not lying at the bottom of a deep channel.

The first test proceeded as planned. A short distance from shore the *Turtle* was lowered into the water. In all of history there was no precedent to show whether David's theories were right or wrong. He was now risking his life to prove that they were right.

Seated on the beam buttressing the sides, David found his eyes on a level with the small windows around the crown of the conning tower. Through them, by the light of the moon, he could see the rippling water of the Sound. Directly above his head, two brass tubes admitted fresh air, and an exhaust ventilator slightly aft of the conning tower ejected stale air.

Inside, everything was within easy reach, so that the operator would have no trouble even in the dark. At David's right hand was the tiller. The rods rotating two of the pairs of oars could be operated either by hand, or by foot on the same principle as a spinning wheel. Beneath his foot was the valve which, when depressed, allowed water to enter for the descent. Close at hand was the lever operating the pump which ejected water for the ascent.

The ballast—nine hundred pounds of lead—was carried beneath the craft. As an additional safety factor, two hundred pounds of this, attached to a chain, could be dropped quickly in case of emergency, allowing the craft to rise swiftly to the surface; this was the original safety weight. It could also be let down forty or fifty feet to serve as an anchor.

Once beneath the surface David methodically tested the various operations. He steered by the compass. He rowed forward and backward. Fifteen minutes passed . . . twenty minutes. When he had been down a half-hour the air began to get dangerously stale. It was time to surface, he knew, but he decided to wait just a few more minutes. He dropped the part of the ballast that served as an anchor, and then raised it. At last, after close to forty-five minutes below, he began working the forcing pump to eject the water, cranking the set of paddles above at the same time. Slowly, steadily, the *Turtle* rose to the surface, and David emerged from the conning tower, triumphant.

He was also close to collapse. It was just as he had feared, he admitted bitterly: he was not strong enough to make further tests. His bitterness was short-lived. Ezra was there, and Ezra was keen to hazard future trials.

The *Turtle* now had been launched successfully. She was a masterpiece of compactness and ingenuity, with every aspect designed for maximum efficiency and safety. And, viewed from the standpoint of that day, she was a nearly miraculous achievement.

Nevertheless, now that it was to be Ezra's life at stake, and not his own, David felt that additional precautions were necessary. Only after several runs on the surface did he permit Ezra to take the craft on a dive, and even then a strong piece of rigging was attached to haul her up in case the pump failed or she became mired in the mud below.

In the beginning David allowed only one person other than Ezra to see the *Turtle*. This was his old friend, Dr. Benjamin Gale of Killingworth. Gale, an inventor himself, had struck up an acquaintance with the famous Benjamin Franklin many years before, and now he kept asking David for permission to write to Dr. Franklin about the *Turtle*. Finally David agreed.

Gale also urged David to request assistance from the Connecticut government, and David gave in on this point, too. Matthew Griswold of Lyme, the deputy governor, inspected the *Turtle* and carried a report back to Governor Trumbull and the Connecticut Council of Safety. The time was not ripe; Connecticut had more demands upon its funds than it could meet. The merit of the *Turtle* was not questioned, but the amount of financial aid offered was negligible. Angrily David refused it; he would risk his own money, little as he had, rather than be beholden for such a trifle.

Despite the cloak of mystery David had attempted to throw over his operations, news of the *Turtle* was beginning to circulate. On August 7, Dr. Gale sent off a letter to Dr. Franklin. "This story may appear Romantic, but thus far is Compleated," he wrote. "Give me Leave to Say, it is all Constructed with Great Simplicity, and upon Principles of Natural Philosophy, and I Conceive is not Equalled by any thing I ever heard of or Saw, Except Dr. Franklins Electrical Experiments."

At the time Gale wrote this letter David was in New Haven with a Mr. Doolittle, a skilled watchmaker and mechanic, supervising the construction of the clockwork mechanism that would operate the mine.

In mid-August, less than three weeks after David's graduation, John Lewis, a tutor at Yale, added the following postscript to a letter to Ezra Stiles, soon to become president of the college:

"This man had invented a machine which is now built and almost perfected, to destroy the fleet in Boston Harbor by an explosion of gunpowder. The machine is constructed so that it can move rapidly twenty or more feet underwater, carrying two thousand pounds of powder to be attached to the hull of a ship. A clockwork will ignite the whole mass either immediately or in half an hour, whichever the operator wishes."

Lewis's report was slightly inaccurate. The *Turtle* was intended to go much farther than twenty feet, and David planned her to carry only a fraction of the two thousand pounds John Lewis spoke of. Lewis at least took the precaution of writing in Latin to preserve some measure of secrecy.

As David expected, these first trials disclosed some problems. Air, for one. When the hatch was secured, the air tubes and ventilator did not function properly. But once David changed the position of the ventilator it drew fresh air through one tube and ejected stale air through the other. To supply more air when the craft was on the surface, he provided three portholes in the conning tower, one each in the front and on the sides, large enough to put the hand through. The shutters of these portholes were ground down with emery to fit perfectly tight.

To prevent the air tubes from being clogged by seaweed or damaged by floating debris, each had a kind of hollow sphere fixed around the top, perforated with holes to allow air to enter. When the vessel submerged, valves in both tubes shut automatically as the water rose near their tops. As a double precaution, caps at the bottom of the tubes could be screwed open or shut by the operator. There was also a perforated plate at the mouth of the water intake tube in the keel, to keep seaweed and fish from slipping in.

One problem continued to plague David. Underwater, with the portholes and air tubes shut, the *Turtle* contained only enough air to support the operator for half an hour. This meant that the operator had to work swiftly and surely when planting the mine, and it placed a dangerous limitation upon the capabilities of the craft. If only some way could be found to provide more air!

Another problem was easily solved. The pair of oars for turning the craft around proved superfluous, so David removed them. At the stem the *Turtle* now had a pair of paddles twelve inches long and about four inches wide to propel the craft forward or backward. A smaller pair, to propel the vessel upward or downward once the craft was submerged (much like hydroplanes), was located a bit forward of the conning tower.

With these modifications made, David let Ezra and the *Turtle* risk deeper channels. Now he had Ezra submerge the *Turtle* and propel her along underwater at various depths. All went smoothly, and the two brothers hastened preparations for the final test, the purpose for which the *Turtle* had been conceived: to attach an underwater mine to the keel of a ship.

To accomplish this, David had provided, close to the conning tower, a socket through which an iron tube passed. The tube could slide up and down six inches. A sharp iron screw, like an auger bit, was attached to the tip of the tube, and from this screw a rod extended down through the tube into the interior. When under a ship, the operator pushed the tube and screw up against the keel, twisted the screw in, and then disengaged the rod, leaving the screw in the planks of the keel.

From this screw a strong rope ran to the powder magazine, or mine. This mine was carried at the stern of the *Turtle*, slightly above the rudder, and was attached to the craft by the same screw which operated as a lock on the works of the clock within the mine. Once this screw was removed, the mine floated free of the *Turtle* and the clockwork mechanism to fire the gunlock and explode the powder was started. The rope, of course, kept the mine beneath the keel of the ship to be blasted.

For the trials, powder was scarce—and so were target ships. David and Ezra made do with dry runs. Speaking of Ezra, David said, "I made him approach a vessel, go under her, and fix the wood-screw in her bottom, until I thought him sufficiently expert to put my design into execution."

Early in October, exciting news arrived. Benjamin Franklin was on his way north from Philadelphia, sent by the Continental Congress to confer with General Washington in Cambridge about reorganizing the Continental Army. And on the way he planned to stop at Killingworth to visit Dr. Gale.

When Franklin arrived, Gale took him over to see the *Turtle*. For David this was a glorious moment. The famous Dr. Franklin, a man he had revered for years, was coming to inspect his invention! Reticent as David was with others, he talked freely about his work to the sixty-nine-year-old Franklin.

Franklin reached Cambridge on October 18, and he may well have been the one who brought word of the *Turtle*'s imminent arrival in camp. Five days after this Samuel Osgood was

41

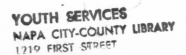

writing excitedly to John Adams about "the famous Water Machine from Connecticutt."

However, there are indications that some hint of the *Turtle*'s mission had arrived earlier—and that it had been passed on to the British commander, General Thomas Gage. In September an American officer in British pay had written to Gage, alluding to a device by which the Americans hoped to destroy the British Navy. Fortunately for David, the spy did not seem to feel that the machine threatened much danger.

Anxious to get the *Turtle* up to Boston as speedily as possible, David decided to make a test with a loaded mine, even though powder was scarce and expensive. He cajoled one of the Saybrook shipowners into giving him an old hulk about to be scuttled, and Ezra—with no way of being sure whether the hulk or the *Turtle* would be blown to pieces—made the attack. The hulk was demolished, Ezra returned safely, and David came away convinced that his mine could hold three times as much powder as was needed to destroy the largest ship in the British Navy.

Early in November Dr. Gale communicated his enthusiasm to Silas Deane, one of the Connecticut delegates at the Continental Congress: "You may call me a visionary, or what you please,—and I do insist upon it, that I believe the inspiration of the Almighty has given him the understanding for this very purpose and design. . . . What astonishment it will produce and what advantages may be made by those on the spot, if it succeeds, is more easy for you to conceive than for me to describe."

Unwittingly, Gale fed information to the British military intelligence. He later discovered that the tavern-keeper and postmaster at Killingworth was a Tory, and that he had opened many of Gale's letters before sending them on.

From this source word of the *Turtle* traveled through the

espionage network set up by the infamous Loyalist and former governor of New York, William Tryon. On November 16, 1775, Tryon sent the following dispatch to Vice Admiral Shuldham: "The great news of the day with us is now to Destroy the Navy, a certain Mr. Bushnel has compleated his Machine, and has been missing four weeks, returned this day week."

"It is conjectur'd," said the report, "that an attempt was made on the *Asia,* but proved unsuccessful—Return'd to New Haven in order to get a Pump of a new Construction which will soon be compleated,—When you may expect to see the Ships in Smoke."

Actually, the report of the spy was in error. Despite the hopes of all concerned, the *Turtle* had not made the trip to Boston. The pump had been giving trouble, and David was not going to risk the craft in action until he was sure she would perform perfectly.

Luckily Shuldham had more on his mind than the report from Tryon, and no immediate attempt was made to seize Bushnell and destroy the *Turtle.*

A week later Dr. Gale wrote again to Silas Deane. "I supposed the machine was gone," he said, "but since find one proving the navigation of it in Connecticut River. The forcing pump made by Mr. Doolittle, not being made according to order given, did not answer; which has delayed him. . . . I suppose he sets off this day with his new constructed pump, in order to prove the navigation, and if not prevented by ice in the River, will proceed soon. . . . He is by no means discouraged in the attempt."

Even the new pump did not answer the needs of the *Turtle.* David was forced to use two pumps before the craft could ascend to the surface swiftly enough.

Then another problem arose, and another delay resulted.

To aid in the navigation of the *Turtle*, David had provided a compass by which the operator could steer his course, a water-gauge to show how deep the *Turtle* was underwater, and a line and lead to sound the depth of the water beneath the craft. The compass and water-gauge caused trouble.

The water-gauge, or barometer, was as ingenious as everything else about the *Turtle*. It was made of a glass tube eighteen inches long and an inch in diameter, standing upright. Its upper end was closed, and its open lower end was struck into a brass pipe through which water entered from outside the submarine. The tube was marked with graduated lines to indicate various depths, and within the tube was a piece of cork. As the submarine descended, the water rose in the tube, condensing the air within, and the cork rose, indicating the depth of the submarine under the water.

The problem was to illuminate both the cork in the water-gauge and the points of the compass so that the operator could see them at night or when the *Turtle* submerged and the interior was thrown into darkness.

At first David tried using fox fire, a wood that glows in the dark. A small piece of this was attached to the cork, and two small pieces in the form of a cross to the north point of the compass. But, as winter came on, he was astonished to discover that frost destroyed the phosphorescent quality of the wood.

In desperation he tried a candle, but its flame consumed the vessel's small supply of oxygen too rapidly. Then David thought of Dr. Franklin. Perhaps he could propose a solution!

During the first week in December Dr. Gale passed the request on to Silas Deane. "The person, the inventor of this machine," Gale wrote, "now makes all his affairs a secret even to his best friends, and I have the liberty to communicate this much from him only with a view to know if Dr. Franklin knows of any kind of phosphorus that will answer his purpose; otherwise the execution must be omitted until next spring, after the frosts are past. I am therefore to request you strictest silence in the matter."

Other worries were besetting David. His own money was about to run out, and he was forced to postpone some of the trials until he could borrow funds from friends. By this time the cold weather which rendered the fox fire useless caused further delays. Now, unless another method of illumination was devised, the *Turtle* would have to sit till spring.

Christmas passed, and then New Year's Day. Early in February Dr. Gale, now mindful of the Tory postmaster at Killingworth, wrote once more to Silas Deane: "With regard to the matter of principal concern, if the Philosopher's Lanthorn may be attained, and will give a better light than what is proposed, should be glad you would get what knowledge you can from Dr. Franklin respecting it. . . . You will well understand my meaning, if I am not more explicit. I have lately seen the man, and conversed freely with him. He is no enthusiast; a perfect philosopher, and by no means doubtful of succeeding."

As Dr. Gale reported, David refused to be discouraged by the difficulties and delays. For one thing, during the cold weather military operations had come nearly to a standstill, and the ice in Boston Harbor made an attack by the *Turtle* impossible. For another thing, David still was convinced that the *Turtle* would operate successfully once the time was ripe.

In the meantime, he set about trying to raise more funds. On February 2, the day after Gale wrote to Deane, David appeared before the Governor of Connecticut and the Connecticut Council of Safety, at their request, and gave an account "of his machine contrived to blow [up] ships."

The Council voted to keep his plans secret and offered to pay the expenses of his journey from Saybrook to Lebanon, Connecticut, where they were meeting. They also voted that "we approve of his plan and that it will be agreeable to have him proceed to make every necessary preparation and experiment about it, with expectation of proper public notice and reward."

The following morning, Saturday, the matter came up again. "It appearing to be a work of great ingenuity," the records noted, "and a prospect that it may be attended with success, and being undertaken merely to serve the public, and of considerable expense to labour &c., it is tho't reasonable that something should be done."

Something was done. On that morning £60 was given to Matthew Griswold "For the use of the Colony. Suppose for Mr. Bushnell, Machine maker." To David, the £60 seemed like a fortune.

VI ➤ The *Turtle* Sets Out

SPRING CAME. Although Dr. Franklin apparently had no solution to the problem of illumination, with spring the fox fire glowed again. David made ready to hustle the *Turtle* up to Boston.

With the spring thaws, the two immobile armies began to stir. Eager for action, the Continentals seized Dorchester Heights, southeast of Boston, and trained their cannons upon the town and the harbor.

Menaced by these batteries, General Howe had no place to go except to sea, and to sea he went. By March 17, 1776, all his troops had embarked upon the transports in the harbor. With the soldiers went more than a thousand Boston Tories— men, women and children—who abandoned everything they owned rather than stay behind to face the tarbrush and feathers, or perhaps worse.

From private to commanding general, the British were glad to be gone. Hell itself, they said, could not afford worse shelter than Boston.

"Whither they are bound, and where they next will pitch their tents," wrote Washington, "I know not." One thing was certain: the thirteen united colonies were not yet free of the British yoke. Washington's hunch was that the enemy would reappear at New York, and as quickly as possible he dispatched

47

most of his troops to start fortifying Manhattan Island.

The streets of New York were, according to John Adams, "vastly more regular and elegant than those in Boston," and the houses "more grand as well as neat," but it was not the grandeur of New York that Washington feared would draw the British: it was the Hudson River.

The Hudson was a passage to the Great Lakes—and to Canada. It was a natural line of defense. By seizing it the British could split the colonies in two. Moreover, the island of Manhattan, surrounded by waters which the Royal Navy could easily penetrate, would make an ideal base from which the British could launch a campaign up the Hudson. The small, ill-equipped American Navy had brave men, but their spirit exceeded their strength, and they were in no position to stop the British.

Washington himself set out for New York on April 4, traveling by way of New London, Lyme and New Haven. On April 11 the General crossed the Connecticut River to Saybrook. According to one story, he spotted the *Turtle*, summoned David Bushnell for a private demonstration, and then urged him to bring the submarine on down to New York. Actually, it appears that the *Turtle* and its inventor did not attract Washington's attention until nearly five months later in a time of violent crisis.

For two months the Americans on Manhattan and Long Island labored in the summer heat to construct fortifications. By now it was known that General Howe and the troop transports were lurking in the waters around Halifax, waiting for reinforcements from England. The target for their attack was still a mystery.

In late June four British men-of-war appeared off Sandy Hook, sailed through the Narrows, and dropped anchor in New York Bay. The next day the lookout on Staten Island gave the alarm: forty sail were in sight. Soon new arrivals swelled the number of ships in the bay to more than a hundred.

As Washington had anticipated, General Howe was swooping down from Halifax. Within a week about ten thousand British soldiers had landed on Staten Island, and the hillsides were white with tents. No movement was made to attack the town of New York or to ascend the Hudson. The affable, self-indulgent Billy Howe was waiting for his elder brother, an admiral, and the more enterprising of the two. At fifty-one, Admiral Lord Richard Howe was dark, cool and resolute. "Give us Black Dick," said one of his sailors, "and we fear nothing."

On July 9 couriers from the Continental Congress in Philadelphia came galloping into New York, bearing copies of the newly adopted Declaration of Independence. At six o'clock that evening the brigades were drawn up to hear the Declaration read aloud. Later that night a mob pulled down the gilded lead statue of King George III that stood in the center of Bowling Green, broke it into pieces, and sent the lead off to be turned into bullets.

Three days later terror took the place of joy.

Everyone with a spyglass had been reconnoitering the bay. About half-past three on the afternoon of July 12 a shout of alarm went up. The 44-gun *Phoenix* and the 20-gun *Rose* came sweeping up the bay, borne on by a fair wind and favorable tide, and proceeded up the Hudson. The fire from the American batteries was almost ludicrously ineffective. The two ships sailed blithely up the Hudson to drop anchor near Tarrytown.

That same evening the Americans found a new reason to be anxious. From the British ships anchored at Staten Island came a great booming of cannon. Through their spyglasses the Americans could see a grand ship-of-the-line, the 64-gun *Eagle*, standing in from sea, with every man-of-war in the British fleet thundering a salute as she passed. From the lookout at the Battery the word flew through New York town: "It is the admiral's ship!" "Black Dick" had come.

Lord Richard Howe had come with every intention of trying to reconcile the rebellious colonies with the mother country, but he arrived too late. The Declaration of Independence had been read from New Hampshire to Georgia; the colonists were not likely to forget it.

The arrival of Admiral Howe made the Americans more desperate than ever to find some scheme to frustrate the British Navy. One of the most ardent schemers was Major General Israel Putnam of Connecticut. Squat and stout, this brave old man had been a military hero long before the Revolution, and his courage at Bunker Hill had become almost a legend. His men followed him with a fanatic devotion. Everyone, even Washington, that stickler for formality, called him "Old Put." Back in Boston, before the movement to New York, one of his officers had written, "Every thing thaws here except Old Put. He is still as hard as ever, crying out 'Powder! powder! ye gods, give me powder!'"

Now, when "Old Put" discovered that the batteries at Fort Washington (between what was later to be 181st Street and 186th Street) had failed to halt the *Phoenix* and the *Rose* on their course up the Hudson, he took steps to stop them whenever they returned.

He set his men to work on a project to obstruct the river channel parallel to Fort Washington and Fort Lee, which was on the Jersey side of the Hudson. This was to be accomplished by means of *chevaux-de-frise*, which were made by sinking wooden beams topped by iron spikes that protruded above the surface of the water. These, it was hoped, would delay the passage of the ships and allow the shore batteries more time to

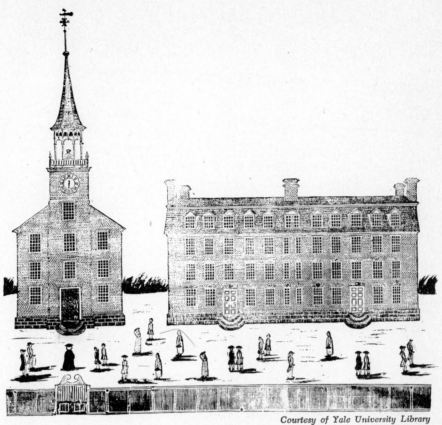

A front view of Yale College and the College Chapel, New Haven

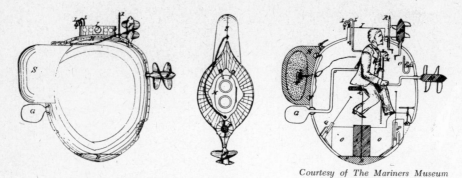

Courtesy of The Mariners Museum

A diagram of the *Turtle* drawn in 1875 by Lieutenant F. M. Barber. His conception of her screw propellers was incorrect.

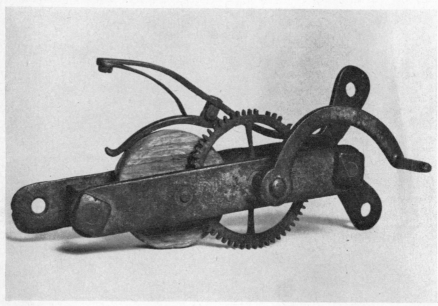

Courtesy of The Submarine Library

A clockwork mechanism believed to have been part of one of David Bushnell's floating mines, now in The Connecticut Historical Society

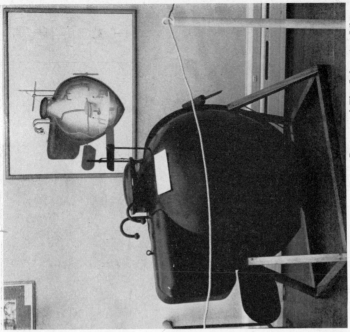

The model of the *Turtle*, built to one-half her original size, in The Submarine Library

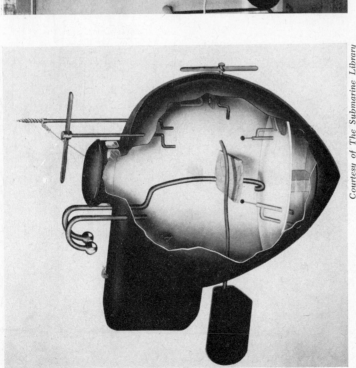

A recent drawing of the *Turtle*, showing the propellers correctly

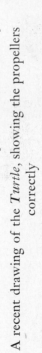

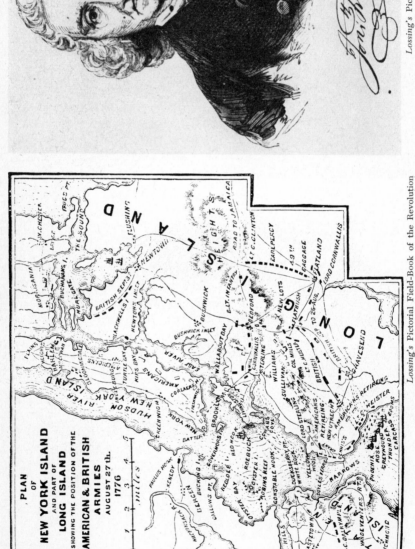

Jonathan Trumbull

Map of New York harbor, 1776

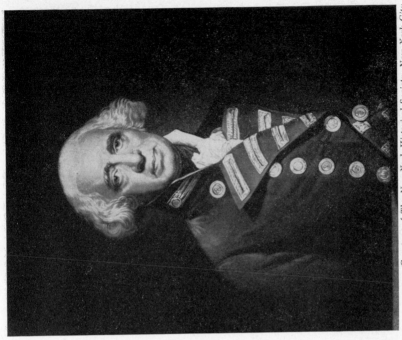

Right Honorable Richard, Earl Howe

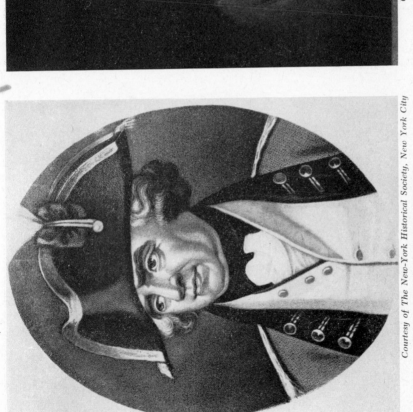

General Sir William Howe

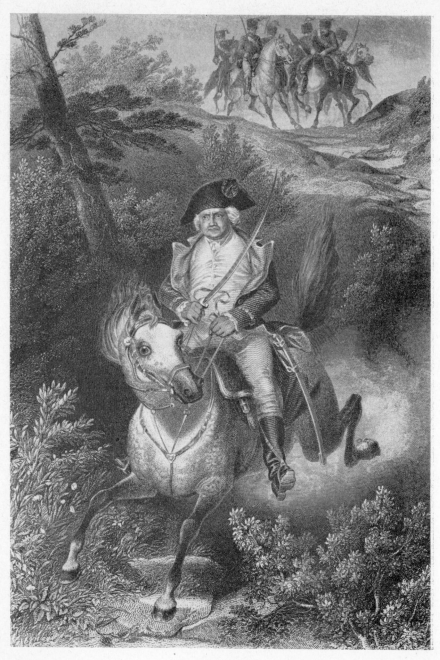

Israel Putnam
From an original drawing by Chappel.

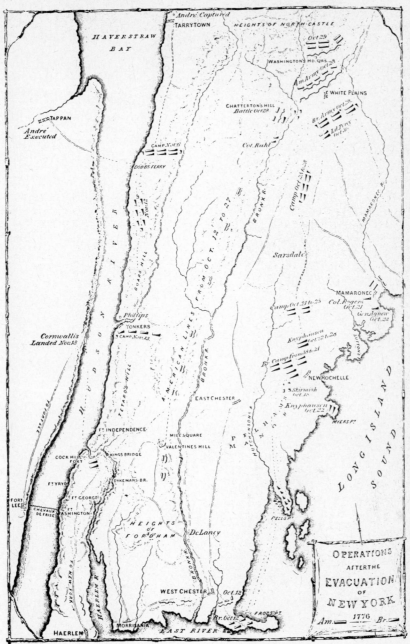

Map of the Hudson River, 1776

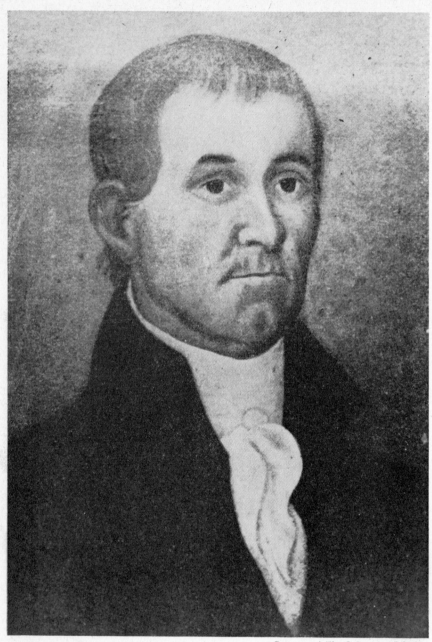

Ezra Lee

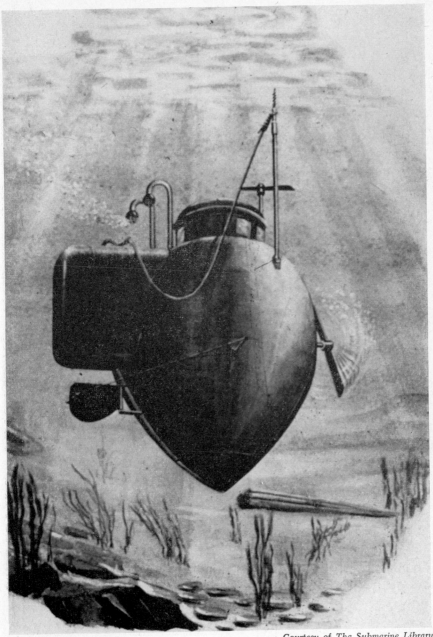

Artist's conception of the *Turtle*

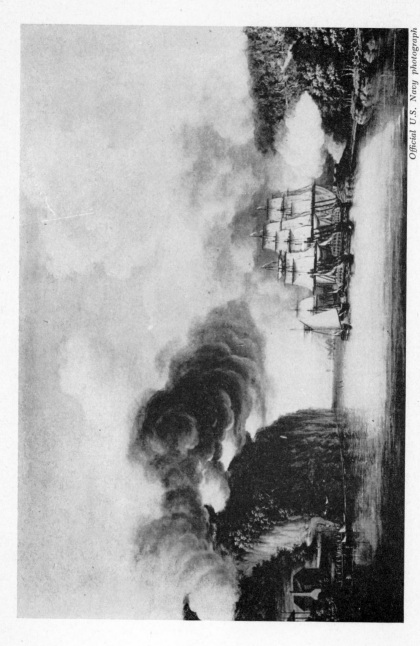

The engagement on the Hudson River, October 9, 1776, during which the *Turtle* was sunk

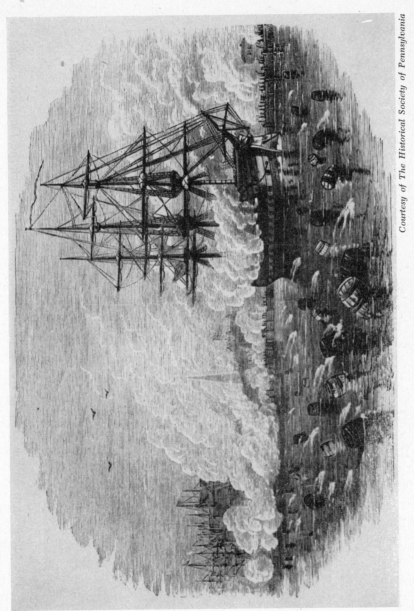

The Battle of the Kegs

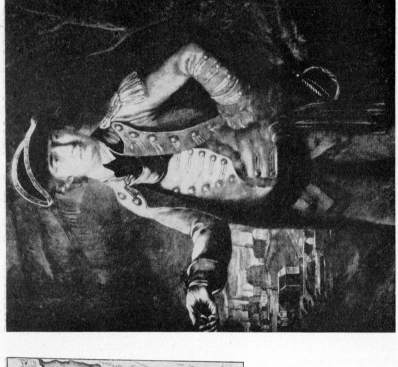

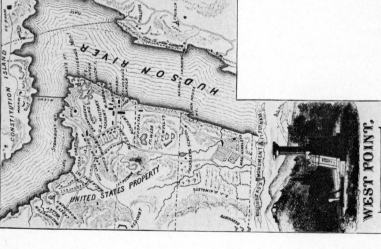

Map of West Point and vicinity

Benedict Arnold

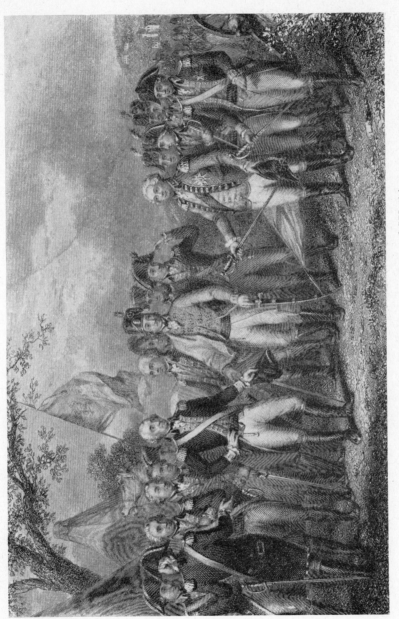

The British surrendering their arms to General Washington, 1781

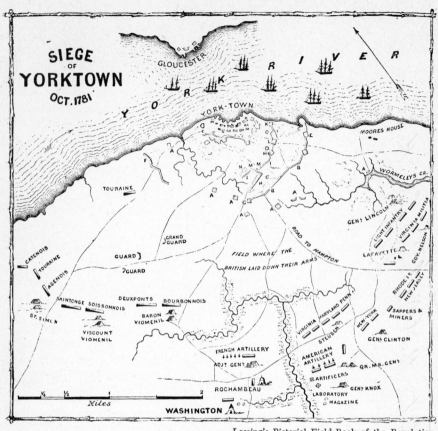

Lossing's Pictorial Field-Book of the Revolution

Map of the siege of Yorktown, 1781

A ration Return for two Men Discharged from the Corps of Sappers & Miners to Carry them to — Conecticut Commencing the fifth & Ending the Eleventh of July 1703 —

	No. of Days	No. of Rations
two Privates	7	14
Total —		14.

Issue one the Above Return — fourteen Rations —

D Bushnell Cap.t Com.t

A ration return bearing David Bushnell's signature

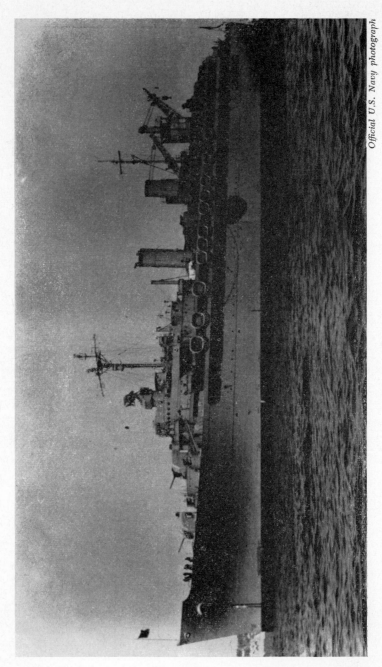

USS *Bushnell* (AS 15)

land their shots.

"We make great despatch," reported Putnam toward the end of July, "by the help of ships, which are to be sunk—a scheme of mine which you may be assured is very simple. . . . The two ships' sterns lie towards each other, about seventy feet apart. Three large logs, which reach from ship to ship, are fastened to them. The two ships and logs stop the river two hundred and eighty feet. The ships are to be sunk, and when hauled down on one side, the pricks will be raised to a proper height, and they must inevitably stop the river, if the enemy will let us sink them."

By early August four ships, chained and boomed, had been scuttled to block the channel.

Then "Old Put" entered zealously upon another scheme, proposed by Ephraim Anderson of one of the Jersey battalions, to build fireships that could be hurled against the enemy shipping to send it up in flames. These craft, deceptively unwarlike in appearance, were loaded with combustibles and smeared with turpentine. Leading to the combustibles were trains of powder which, when lit, would act as a fuse. "We are preparing fourteen fireships to go into their fleet," Putnam wrote, "some of which are ready charged and fitted to sail, and I hope soon to have them all fixed."

Meanwhile, British ships had continued to pour into the bay, ships with a thousand Hessians, ships with Scotch Highlanders, ships with Sir Henry Clinton and Lord Cornwallis and three thousand troops recently repulsed at Charleston, South Carolina. By now the harbor was so crowded with masts that one observer said the bay looked like a pine forest with all the branches trimmed.

The assembled force of the enemy was more than thirty thousand. The Continentals had less than twenty thousand, of which one-fourth were on the sick list with fevers and dysentery, and the rest were scattered over far-distant posts and out-posts. Any means of putting a stop to the British Navy and the Howe brothers was desperately needed.

"Where is Bushnel?" complained William Williams, a member of the Continental Congress, writing to his brother-in-law, Colonel Joseph Trumbull. "Why dont he attempt something when will or can be a more proper Time than is or has been etc I was knowing to his coming etc and that you was acquainted with the Plan etc."

Since Colonel Trumbull was Commissary General of the Continental Army as well as the son of the Governor of Connecticut, it would seem that David's attempt to get the *Turtle* into action was gaining high-ranking support.

But it was still David's attempt. The Continental forces were shockingly disorganized, and Washington's efforts to set matters straight were hampered by the muddling of Congress. As a result, the military tended to act with an independence that seems almost incredible today. If the *Turtle* saw action, it would be thanks to David Bushnell's energy, determination and sheer audacity. There was no efficient military machine to smooth the approaches to his target. The army might help, but the responsibility would be David's.

On a sloop borrowed from one of the shipowners in Saybrook or New London, David and Ezra managed to get the *Turtle* down to the vicinity of New York. Now that the fox fire would light the compass, David felt that the *Turtle* was safe and seaworthy. Even more important, by now Ezra was, according to David, "very ingenious and [has] made himself master of the business."

"He came to me in 1776, recommended by Governor Trumbull and other respectable characters, who were converts to his plan," George Washington wrote to Thomas Jefferson nine years later. "Although I wanted faith myself, I furnished him with money and other aids to carry his plan into execution."

Others were more enthusiastic. David Humphreys, then serving as a volunteer adjutant, for one. And "Old Put" for another.

When news of the *Turtle*'s arrival reached Putnam, he sent one of his aides to interview Bushnell and inspect the submarine. This aide, a handsome young man of twenty years, was something of a dandy, though he had distinguished himself earlier while serving under Benedict Arnold. He was as anxious as Putnam to find a way to thwart the British. Just a few days before being sent to Bushnell, he had written his uncle, "They hold us in the utmost contempt. Talk of forcing all our lines without firing a gun. The bayonet is their pride. They have forgot Bunker's Hill."

This young man, Aaron Burr, apparently brought back a favorable report; Putnam soon was supporting the *Turtle* as ardently as any of the earlier projects intended to harass the British fleet. He had good reason: the other schemes were not doing well.

On the night of August 17 two of the recently constructed fireships set off up the Hudson River to attack the *Phoenix* and the *Rose*, which had been alarming the countryside around Tarrytown. The first of the fireships, in making for the *Rose*, encountered one of her tenders instead, yet did manage to leave the small boat in flames. Although the other fireship succeeded in grappling the *Phoenix*, in the darkness the ship got to the leeward of the man-of-war and was cut loose before any damage could be done.

As if to show a haughty contempt for the American efforts, early the next morning the *Phoenix* and the *Rose*, taking advantage of a brisk wind, sailed down the river. Reaching Fort Washington, they kept close in to the shore, where the batteries of the fort could not be brought to bear. The *chevaux-de-frise* might just as well not have been built. One small passage through them had been left open. This the *Phoenix* and the *Rose* discovered. They sailed through and on down toward the bay, without suffering any apparent damage.

Putnam's support seemed almost a jinx to any venture he supported, for about this time a calamity overtook the *Turtle*.

Ezra Bushnell, who had been navigating the *Turtle* for nearly a year—and was the only man trained to operate her—was stricken with the fever that had laid low so many of the soldiers in the Continental Army. He would be out of action for weeks. The tempo of the war was quickening. Where would David find a replacement?

Washington himself summed up the quandary: "It was no easy matter to get a person hardy enough to encounter the variety of dangers, to which he would be exposed; first, from the novelty; secondly, from the difficulty of conducting the machine, and governing it under water, on account of the current; and thirdly, from the consequent uncertainty of hitting the object devoted to destruction, without rising frequently above water for fresh observations, which, when near the vessel, would expose the adventurer to discovery and to almost certain death."

All the intense, careful training Ezra had undergone was wasted. The future of the *Turtle* was now in jeopardy. If no volunteer could be found—or if none of the volunteers proved skillful enough—the whole project would have to be abandoned.

For several days David had no luck in his frantic search for volunteers. Then, probably at the suggestion of "Old Put," he went to Brigadier General Samuel Parsons, who was under Putnam's command. Parsons, who hailed from Lyme, headed a brigade of Connecticut troops. As one of the volunteers later reported, David put in an appeal for "some one to go learn the ways and mystery of this new machine and to make a trial of it."

Parsons immediately sent for three men who had submitted their names to man a fireship if needed. One of these was his brother-in-law, Ezra Lee, a twenty-seven-year-old sergeant.

Sergeant Lee and the two others agreed to take the risk. Although David was pessimistic about their ability to master the operation of the *Turtle* in a short time, he was unwilling to give up without a try. A year of hard work, several years of planning, and all his money had gone into the invention.

With the *Turtle* loaded aboard a sloop, David and his three volunteers proceeded down Long Island Sound. Along the way they stopped at various small inlets and harbors with which the north shore of the Sound abounds. There David gave the three novices preliminary training. They dared not stop for long in any one spot. The network of spies organized by Governor Tryon of New York was still very active, and there was always danger of betrayal by a stray Tory.

Even more ominous, there was constant danger of surprise by the British. At any moment a man-of-war might descend upon them, sink the *Turtle*, and kill or imprison the little band undertaking this desperate mission. Worse still, the *Turtle* herself might fall into British hands, to be turned against the American ships.

Finally the *Turtle* reached the Connecticut River and Saybrook. Here trials could be conducted with greater safety. David was familiar with the conditions. So was Sergeant Lee, having grown up at Lyme. David now made what were described as "some little alterations" in the machinery, no doubt as the result of small imperfections discovered in the trials along

55

the Sound.

This trip back to Saybrook had taken about ten days. In the meantime, the situation for the Continental Army at New York had changed drastically. The storm had been gathering. Now it broke.

VII ➤ "That'll Do It for 'em!"

ON THURSDAY morning, August 22, 1776, Sir William Howe landed about ten thousand troops on Long Island, and although Israel Putnam was immediately dispatched to head the American resistance, the British swept forward, sending smoke from their rifles and cannons high above the orchards and groves. Fighting fiercely every foot of the way, the Continentals were pushed back to the heights of Brooklyn, leaving Washington no alternative but to evacuate Long Island and retreat to Manhattan.

For the escape, boats were mustered by John Glover of Marblehead, heading an heroic band of sailors and fishermen. From midnight on August 29, until the following dawn, boat after boat, their oars muffled and their movements cloaked by a dense fog, carried troops, artillery, ammunition, provisions, cattle, horses and carts to safety on Manhattan, unloading them at the wharves from Fulton Ferry to Whitehall. Except for a few pieces of heavy artillery, almost everything was salvaged from the debacle.

While the Americans were bringing off this near miracle, "the high-feeding English general slept on," said an Englishman, "and his brother the admiral did not move a single ship or boat, and was to all appearances unconscious of what was going on."

The Americans found little joy in the way the Battle of Long Island had ended. They had lost about fifteen hundred men, including those taken prisoner, nearly five times the losses of the British. That very night a 40-gun ship sailed up the East River to Turtle Bay, a small, rock-bound cove at the foot of what is now East 44th to 47th Streets; and Admiral Howe moved the rest of his fleet up New York Bay to anchor near Governor's Island.

The American troops were riddled by fear, despair and disgust. Many of them felt a strong desire to go home, and home they went—by whole regiments, by half ones, and by companies at a time. In a few days the Connecticut militia dwindled from six or eight thousand to less than two thousand.

North along the Boston Post Road couriers bore word of the defeat. When the news reached Saybrook, David Bushnell made ready to rush the *Turtle* and the three volunteers back to Manhattan. If the *Turtle* did not see action now, she might never have another opportunity. Hustled aboard a sloop, the *Turtle* was carried swiftly down Long Island Sound to New Rochelle, where she was loaded on a cart and hauled overland to the East River. But with the British ship at Turtle Bay, she could not move straight down the river to the tip of Manhattan.

Early in September Brigadier General Parsons wrote an urgent letter to Major General William Heath, then in command at King's Bridge, not far from the Hudson above Fort Washington:

Sir:—

As the machine designed to attempt blowing up the enemy's ships is to be transferred from the East to the North River, where a small vessel will be wanted to receive it, I wish you would order one for the purpose. As all things are now ready to make the experiment, I wish it may not be delayed. Though the event is uncertain, the experiment under our present circumstances is certainly worth trying.

I am, Sir, your obedient
humble servant,
Sam'l H. Parsons

The small vessel was waiting, and on Friday, September 6, the *Turtle* was brought down the Hudson and North Rivers to the southern tip of Manhattan. There it was secured, at Whitehall Battery at the South Ferry Landing, where two 32-pounders menaced the British fleet.

The attempt was to wait for the first favorable night; in a strong tide or swelling seas the *Turtle* tended to be difficult to manage. "Old Put," highly optimistic about the chances of success, announced that he planned to be a spectator whenever the trial was made. Adjutant Davie Humphreys was equally ardent. The *Turtle*, Humphreys said, was "altogether different from anything hitherto devised by the art of man." And, he added, "the simplicity, yet combination discovered in the mechanism of this wonderful machine, were not less ingenious than novel."

The very first night that the *Turtle* lay at Whitehall Battery seemed favorable for the attempt. The waters of the bay were calm, and the ebb tide—to all appearances—was not very strong. Now David had to make the crucial choice: which of the volunteers was to man the *Turtle* on her first mission against the enemy? The man he selected, he said, "appeared more expert than the rest." This was Sergeant Ezra Lee.

The target was to be the mightiest ship in sight: the *Eagle*, Admiral Richard Howe's 64-gun flagship, with "Black Dick" himself aboard.

A tight net of secrecy was drawn around every detail of the mission. Only a handful of men knew of the proposed attack, and shortly before midnight they gathered at the wharf at Whitehall. "Old Put" was there, and probably Davie Humphreys, and perhaps Aaron Burr and Samuel Parsons as well. Although rumors have persisted that Washington was on hand, none of the eyewitness accounts mentioned his presence, and Washington himself never indicated that he was there.

As the *Turtle* bobbed in the water at the foot of the wharf, the mine was placed in position over the rudder. Then a line was run from it to the screw that was to be driven into the wooden keel of the *Eagle*. For several hours the *Turtle* was checked and rechecked, to be sure every safety precaution had been taken. Finally Sergeant Lee clambered aboard, squeezed through the narrow entry, pulled the hatch shut, and fastened it tight. The crews of two whaleboats made ready to tow the strange contraption out into the bay.

"We set off from the city," wrote Sergeant Lee afterwards. "The whale boats towed me as nigh the ships as they dared to go and then cast me off."

Sergeant Lee was now on his own, bobbing up and down in New York Bay in a perilous craft. His training had been brief and hectic, and he had not yet had a chance to learn all the *Turtle*'s quirks. Because of his inexperience, he miscalculated the pull of the tide, which swept him down the bay past the ships.

"I however hove about and rowed for 5 glasses by the ships' bell," Lee said, "before the tide slacked, so that I could get alongside of the man of war which lay above the transports."

Lee had been late in setting off from the wharf. Now two-and-a-half more hours had been wasted, and every moment was precious. By the time he got back on target, the first glow of dawn was beginning to appear on the horizon. There was still enough light from the moon to guide him, but not enough to betray his progress to any casual lookout. Lee felt fairly safe from discovery. None of the sentinels aboard the British ships had been alerted that a submarine was making for the flagship. Indeed, none of them even dreamed that a submarine existed.

At last he came abreast of the *Eagle*. Only six or seven inches of the conning tower protruded above the waves, so no one on deck noticed the weird, log-like object floating close to the side of the ship. As Lee rowed under the stern, the windows in the top and sides of the *Turtle* allowed him a glimpse of the sailors moving about on deck. He had the portholes open to admit air, and through them drifted the voices of the British tars, chatting softly in the early dawn.

Making fast the portholes, he prepared to submerge. A slight pressure of his foot on the valve in the bottom started the water flowing in. He revolved the upper set of oars to speed the descent. Knowing his air supply would last only a half-hour, he worked with feverish haste.

Now to plant the mine. Carefully he pushed up the rod with the screw on the end, the screw to which the line bearing the mine was attached. But something was wrong. There should have been no difficulty in making the screw enter the wooden keel. Even if the keel were sheathed in copper (as some were), the screw should have penetrated; David Bushnell had foreseen this possibility.

But the screw was not entering. Lee could tell that as he twisted the rod. Indeed, each time he pressed the rod against the ship's bottom, the *Turtle* seemed to rebound.

He and David later decided that the screw must have struck the iron bar connecting the rudder hinge with the stern. "Had he moved a few inches," David once wrote, "which he might have done, without rowing, I have no doubt he would have found wood where he might have fixed the screw; or if the ship were sheathed with copper, he might easily have pierced it."

With his hasty training, Sergeant Lee was not as skilled at handling the *Turtle* as Ezra Bushnell would have been. As he pulled along to try again, he deviated a little to one side. With tremendous velocity the *Turtle* shot up to the surface. Lee found himself to the east of the ship, only two or three feet away from the hull, exposed to the spreading light of dawn and in immediate danger of discovery. Desperately he pressed the water valve. As smoothly as a porpoise, the *Turtle* sank again.

"I hove about to try again," Lee later wrote, "but on further thought I gave out, knowing that as soon as it was light the ships' boats would be rowing in all directions, and I thought the best generalship was to retreat as fast as I could, as I had 4 miles to go before Governor's Island. So jogg'd on as fast as I could."

As he jogged along, another accident befell him. Something went wrong with the compass, and with no means of knowing the direction in which he was headed—other than by keeping on the lookout—he dared not submerge. Cranking the set of oars at the stem with one hand, guiding the tiller with the other, he kept the *Turtle* moving along on the surface, with the portholes open. Apparently Lee was shorter than David, for as he perched on the seat, the portholes were too high for him to see out of them properly. Every few moments he had to rise up and crane his neck to make sure he was heading back toward Manhattan—and not toward the British camp on Long Island.

Governor's Island, held by the British, loomed up ahead. To avoid running aground on its shore, Lee steered a crooked, zigzag course.

"When I was abreast of the fort on the Island," he wrote,

"3 or 400 men got upon the parapet to observe me; at leangth a number came down to the shore, shoved off a 12 oar'd barge with 5 or 6 sitters and pulled for me. I eyed them, and when they had got within 50 or 60 yards of me I let loose the magazine in hopes that if they should take me they would likewise pick up the magazine, and then we should all be blown up together."

When Lee cast the mine adrift, the clockwork mechanism to fire the gunlock started ticking. In exactly sixty minutes it was set to explode. However, when the oarsmen spotted the queer cask that had suddenly bobbed up to the surface, they suspected a Yankee trick, took fright, and rowed frantically back to Governor's Island—to Sergeant Lee's infinite relief.

On the *Turtle* moved, against the tide and a considerable swell, until finally Lee came within sight of the anxious group waiting at the wharf at Whitehall. When he signaled, a whaleboat came out and towed him in to shore. He had been afloat in the *Turtle* for about five hours. Though close to exhaustion from the strain of rowing, he had come back alive.

About twenty minutes after Lee had clambered out of the *Turtle* and staggered onto the wharf, while "Old Put" and David Bushnell and the others were listening avidly to the details of his mission, the mine exploded. With tremendous violence it threw a vast column of water and pieces of wood to an amazing height in the air.

"That'll do it for 'em!" Putnam shouted joyfully.

Crowds of soldiers and civilians rushed out of the houses in the neighborhood, startled from their beds by the terrible blast. Because the mission had been so closely guarded, speculation was rampant as to what had caused the ear-shattering roar. A meteor, some said. Or a waterspout. Or an earthquake.

Few suspected that the explosion had come close to signaling

63

the end of the proud *Eagle* and of Admiral Lord Richard Howe.

Aboard the *Eagle* and the other ships in the British fleet, a madhouse of confusion and alarm burst forth when the great column of water was hurled up into the air. Not knowing exactly what was afoot, but suspecting a dire calamity, the British cut their cables instantly, and in great disorder drifted down the bay with the ebbing tide, dropping anchor only when they reached a safe distance. For once, British complacency was badly shaken. They had a major coup planned —a death blow to the American cause, they hoped—and the sinking of the *Eagle*, Lord Howe, and other men-of-war would have caused disastrous delay.

David Bushnell was furious over his bad luck. The *Turtle* had functioned almost perfectly; the mine had exploded right on time. It was only the human factor that had let him down —the human factor and a series of unpredictable accidents. If his brother had not been taken sick and had been able to attack the fleet before the Battle of Long Island . . . if there had been more time to train Sergeant Lee and the others . . . if Lee had left earlier, and not been exposed to danger by the rising sun . . . if the tide had not carried him past the ship . . . if the screw had not struck the iron bar . . . if . . . if . . . if. . . .

David had one prime cause for regret. Sergeant Lee, he wrote, "says that he could easily have fastened the magazine under the stern of the ship, above water, as he rowed up to the stern, and touched it before he descended. Had he fastened it there, the explosion of 150 pounds of powder (the quantity contained in the magazine) must have been fatal to the ship." But Lee had not done this, and the *Eagle* was riding safely at anchor in the lower bay.

David could not be harsh with Lee. After all, he was unskilled, and his instructions had been to attempt to place the mine beneath the ship, and he had done as ordered. Moreover, he had proved beyond doubt that the *Turtle* was no suicide craft. She had stayed afloat, she had submerged—and ascended—properly, and she had brought Sergeant Lee back to shore.

One more chance. Just one more chance, and the *Turtle* would bring off her mission. David was convinced of that. A little more training for the volunteers, and then another attempt at the first favorable moment.

But in the next few days it began to look as if there would be no further chance—for the *Turtle* or for the American Army.

VIII ➤ The *Turtle* Attacks Again
. . . and Again

FIVE DAYS after the *Turtle* just missed sending "Black Dick" Howe to the bottom of New York Bay, Washington decided not to attempt to hold New York against a British invasion. A withdrawal to the hilly northern part of Manhattan Island began at once. To provide cover for the retreating forces, "Old Put," with four or five thousand men, was left temporarily in the town proper at the very southern tip of the island. Samuel Parsons' brigade was one of two stationed at Kip's Bay, a cove on the East River at the foot of today's 34th Street.

The next day, just after dinner, four frigates moved up the East River toward Hell Gate, cannonading the shore as they passed. Three overly curious spectators were killed with one ball. Another landed within six feet of General Washington, who was riding by on horseback. At sunset on Saturday, September 14, these ships were joined by six more, and detachments of British troops began occupying the islands at the mouth of the Harlem River.

Orders to evacuate came before David Bushnell and the *Turtle* could make another attempt to blow up the *Eagle*. The submarine was hoisted aboard a sloop by a "crane" galley

66

and rushed up the North River and the Hudson to Fort Washington—just in time to escape a blockade.

Before very long the notorious 64-gun *Asia* and several other vessels sailed up the Hudson River to anchor opposite Bloomingdale, not far below Fort Washington. At this point Washington was greatly concerned about the security of the Hudson, but he placed great faith in the *chevaux-de-frise*, the obstructions Putnam had built across the river at Fort Washington.

As an additional defense, there were four galleys mounted with heavy guns and swivels to fire upon any enemy ship that tried to break through the obstructions. At hand were two new ships, loaded with stones, which were to be sunk to make the *chevaux-de-frise* more effective. Batteries on each shore, at Fort Lee and at Fort Washington, commanded the obstructions. The Americans were confident that no hostile ship could succeed in passing.

Also present were some fireships. At two o'clock one morning, Captain Silas Talbot and a small crew piloted one of these incendiary vessels down from Fort Washington toward the enemy ships anchored opposite Bloomingdale. Although Talbot did manage to bring his blazing ship alongside the *Asia* and then escape alive to the Jersey shore, he was more severely burned than the man-of-war.

Meanwhile, on the other side of the island, the patriots had their hands full. About eleven o'clock on Sunday morning, September 15, the redcoats led by Sir Henry Clinton landed at Kip's Bay. The American troops stationed there—including Parsons' brigade—fled in panic, despite every attempt by their officers to make them stand their ground. General Washington, galloping up on horseback, tried to rally the panic-stricken men. When his efforts proved futile, he dashed his hat on the ground and raged at the cowards, threatening them with his sword. He was so heedless of his own danger that the enemy troops were within eighty yards before one of his aides seized the bridle of his horse and drew him away to safety.

Down at the southern tip of the island, Israel Putnam received orders to abandon the town. The heat was blistering, yet the old general rode tirelessly back and forth, keeping order among his men as they retreated up the Bloomingdale Road toward safety on the heights of Harlem. By good fortune Major Aaron Burr, who knew every inch of the terrain, was on hand to guide the troops through the unfamiliar ground. Also, by good fortune, Howe, Clinton and several other British officers delayed to have cakes and Madeira sherry at Mrs. Robert Murray's home at Incleberg, now Murray Hill. Howe's battle plan called for a wait while the beachhead was built up, and whether Mrs. Murray was an ardent patriot—intentionally causing the British to linger longer than they had planned—or simply a gracious hostess remains in question.

The next morning, a short distance in front of Harlem Heights, the Connecticut Rangers, a choice regiment known as Congress's Own and commanded by Colonel Knowlton, managed to repulse an attack by the British. Mortally wounded in the battle, Knowlton died before telling Washington that he had sent one of his captains, Nathan Hale, on an espionage mission behind enemy lines.

Their spirits revived by the courage of the Connecticut Rangers, the Americans now began to entrench on the narrow neck of rocky land at the northwestern point of Manhattan Island, bounded on the east and north by the Harlem River and Spyt den Duivel Kill (Spite the Devil Creek) and on the west by the Hudson River. On one of these rocky heights was Fort Washington, where the *Turtle* had sought safety.

Eager to get the *Turtle* back in action, David concentrated on giving Sergeant Lee and the other two navigators more training, although he never abandoned hope that Ezra Bushnell might recover in time to propel the submarine to glory.

The night of September 20 a strong wind was blowing from the southwest. Shortly after midnight the small band at Fort Washington, looking south toward New York, saw broad arrows of flame shooting up, lighting up the dark sky. All night long the fire raged. By dawn one-eighth of the buildings in the town of New York were smoking ruins. Although blame for the holocaust was never fixed, for years recriminations flew back and forth between the British and Americans.

Meanwhile, disguised as a schoolmaster, Captain Nathan Hale of Congress's Own had passed over to Long Island and made his way to the British camp at Brooklyn. There he sketched the fortifications, jotted down notes in Latin, and began his stealthy return toward the American lines. Then his luck ran out. He was recognized, denounced, stripped and searched. Hidden in the soles of his boots the drawings and notes were discovered.

On Saturday, September 21, when the embers still were smoldering in New York, Hale was carried before General Howe, who had taken up quarters in James Beekman's mansion at Turtle Bay. That night Hale was confined in the greenhouse on the Beekman grounds. The next morning, without a trial, he was handed over to William Cunningham, the brutal provost-marshal, for execution. Cunningham refused Hale permission to see a clergyman or to have a Bible and confiscated the two letters he wrote. "The rebels shall not know," swore Cunningham, "that they have a man in their army who can die with so much firmness." That Sunday morning, in the artillery park, Nathan Hale was hanged.

Despite Cunningham, Nathan Hale's last words were later carried to the American camp by a British officer present at the execution. So the rebels did learn of the firmness with which he died: "I only regret that I have but one life to lose for my country."

The news of Nathan Hale's death was a profound shock to David Bushnell and his other friends in the army around New York. The good fellow from the happy days at Yale, the young man with a brilliant future, was gone. They were about the only ones who mourned him. The army as a whole took slight notice at this time. He was just one of many casualties.

These were uneasy days at Fort Washington. As he had not enlisted in the army, David shared few of the scanty benefits of the soldiers—and all of their hardships. He and the *Turtle* had to fend for themselves, and the peril of the situation seemed to be increasing. There was talk that the northwest point of Manhattan could not be held. There was more talk of retreating to White Plains. And there was a constant threat from the three ships now anchored off Bloomingdale—the *Phoenix* and the *Roebuck*, each of 44 guns, and the *Tartar* of 20 guns.

Even though there had been little time or opportunity to give Sergeant Lee and the other two volunteers more training, David decided to send the *Turtle* into action again. He was, in a sense, the commander of his own task force. He planned the strategy, worked out the tactics. If cooperation was forthcoming from the army, fine. If not, he proceeded on his own. He had serious reservations about Lee's abilities, yet the sergeant was undoubtedly the most skilled of the three.

According to Lee, the plan of attack called for him to approach one of the frigates and attach the mine at the stern close to the water's edge. In the raid on the *Eagle* a few weeks back, he had tried to place the mine beneath the keel, even though his best chance had been when he was at the stern.

Setting off from Fort Washington, Sergeant Lee managed to bring the *Turtle* alongside the stern of the frigate without mishap. But the sentinel on watch was alert. Spotting the strange piece of brass moving faster than the tide—obviously not just drifting by—he gave the alarm.

Cooped up in the *Turtle*, Lee heard the hue and cry. No time now to attach the screw and line holding the mine. Securing the portholes and pressing the valve to flood the keel, he frantically cranked the upper set of paddles to hasten the descent. Without a moment to spare the *Turtle* sank beneath the surface, disappearing from view before the sailors aboard the frigate had the presence of mind to begin a bombardment.

Having moved away to a safe distance, Lee surfaced and waited till the commotion died down. Then he decided to try another approach and attach the mine beneath the keel.

At this point, so Lee reported, the barometer stopped working. The position of the cork in the glass tube showed how deep the *Turtle* was descending, but somehow—perhaps because the pipe feeding water to the tube had become clogged—the cork stuck. Lee had no idea how far down he was going. In the confusion he descended too deep and was unable to reach the bottom of the keel with the rod holding the screw. Discouraged by this, shaken by the harrowing experience he had undergone, he abandoned the attempt, moved away from the frigate, and surfaced. Then he paddled back to safety.

David's version of what happened is slightly different. He maintained that Lee miscalculated his distance when approaching the frigate and went so far beyond that he lost sight of her.

"When he at last found her," said David, "the tide ran so strong, that as he descended under water, for the ship's bottom—it swept him away."

Once again, if Ezra Bushnell had been on hand, the results might have been different. By now David was close to physical collapse. "I had been in a bad state of health from the beginning of my undertaking," he later said, "and was now very unwell." However, he urged a third attack, which was made a day or so later, this time with another of the volunteers. This mission, as David tersely put it, "effected nothing."

Lack of time and lack of money were pressing him hard, and Ezra gave no indication of recovering sufficiently to navigate the *Turtle*. "I found it absolutely necessary," David said, "that the operators should acquire more skill in the management of the vessel, before I could expect success." But this, he added, "would have taken up some time, and made no small additional expense."

The decision was taken out of his hands. At eight o'clock on the morning of October 9, a few days after the *Turtle*'s third attack, an easy southern breeze was blowing. The *Phoenix*, *Roebuck* and *Tartar*, the ships that had been lying opposite Bloomingdale, now hauled up anchor and sailed up the Hudson toward Fort Washington.

There a pitiable American fleet huddled—the two ships loaded with stones for the *chevaux-de-frise*, as well as four galleys and a schooner with a cargo of rum, sugar and supplies for the Continental Army. Here, too, was the sloop bearing David Bushnell, Sergeant Lee and the *Turtle*.

As the *Phoenix*, *Roebuck* and *Tartar* approached, the American craft fled before the breeze. The British moved steadily on toward the *chevaux-de-frise*, apparently oblivious to the constant fire from seven batteries on the shore. One lookout reported that a gentleman was walking the deck of the *Phoenix* as calmly as if he were out for a morning stroll. Actually, considerable damage was done to their masts and rigging; a lieutenant, two midshipmen and six men were killed; and eighteen were wounded.

Almost like cutting a cobweb, the *Phoenix, Roebuck* and *Tartar* sailed through the *chevaux-de-frise,* and the American vessels scudded fearfully before them. Two of the galleys found haven in a cove, but the schooner laden with supplies was overhauled and captured, and the two ships loaded with stones were driven ashore at Phillips' Mills at Yonkers.

The British continued hard in pursuit of the other two galleys. As the breeze freshened, they gained, raining grapeshot on the fugitives. At one-thirty in the afternoon the hunters drove their prey ashore at Dobbs' Ferry. Some of the enemy then landed at the hamlet and plundered a store before setting fire to it.

What of the sloop bearing the *Turtle?* At about ten o'clock that sunny Wednesday morning in October, a well-aimed shot had sent her—and the *Turtle*—to the bottom of the river. David, Sergeant Lee and the others swam to safety on the shore, as the *Turtle* settled into the mud of the Hudson River bed. "Its fate," said General William Heath, "was truly a contrast to its design."

But so far as David was concerned, the *Turtle* had not yet met her fate. He managed to recruit a crew to salvage the submarine—no mean feat considering the chaos that reigned at Fort Washington and the perils of the undertaking.

"Though I afterwards recovered the vessel," he wrote, "I found it impossible, at that time, to prosecute the design any farther." And he had good reason to call a temporary halt. "The situation of public affairs was such," he explained, "that I despaired of obtaining the public attention, and the assistance necessary. I was unable to support myself, and the persons I must have employed."

Money . . . there was always the problem of money. And the problem of men. As a volunteer, almost a guerrilla, he found the path riddled with pitfalls. Even so, he had no intention of abandoning the *Turtle*. He merely was waiting, he said, "for a more favorable opportunity."

IX ➤ "Their Secret Modes
of Mischief"

BEFORE THE more favorable opportunity arrived, a maelstrom threatened to engulf the patriots. Within three weeks of the sinking—and salvage—of the *Turtle,* the Continental forces were defeated at White Plains. Then Fort Washington and Fort Lee fell, and General Washington began a retreat across New Jersey toward Pennsylvania.

David made his way back to the Bushnell farm in Saybrook. What became of the *Turtle* remains a mystery. When he was forced to flee from Fort Washington, David may have dismantled her and destroyed the parts, to keep her from the hands of the British. It would have been a bitter irony to see her put to work against the Continental Navy. And a new— and better—*Turtle* could be built later, if he could scrape together the money.

Or the *Turtle* may have been carted back to the Pochaug farm and hidden in the barn, awaiting a new opportunity to venture forth on a raid. But after the autumn of 1776 she never saw action again. No record has survived to indicate what fate she finally met. The first submarine in history to take the offensive against an enemy ship seemed simply to disappear.

David was not daunted by the troubles the *Turtle* had met.

He already had another project in mind, and soon after returning to Saybrook he was at work upon it. For a one-man task force—himself—the submarine had involved too much expense, too many problems, too much dependence upon the assistance of others. Since that was so, he would devise a simpler plan, one that would make use of his underwater mine. The mine, of course, had been his original device, and the *Turtle* herself had been created mainly as a way to carry the mine to the target. Now he was determined to improve the mine so that it could reach and demolish its target in a different manner.

As David labored through the winter to make new improvements in his mine, the war dispatches from south of Connecticut brought little cheer. Although Washington had managed to brake the retreat of his army, recross the Delaware, occupy Trenton and defeat the British at Princeton, the cold weather brought his campaign to a halt. The army was forced into winter encampment at Morristown, New Jersey, and from Morristown came letters telling of fierce privation and suffering.

David knew the dangers under which he worked. In both New York and Rhode Island, the British seemed poised to spring upon Connecticut at any moment. Redcoats seemed to be everywhere, and British spies as well. More and more reports circulated about spies who had been apprehended and hanged. A favorite story concerned Israel Putnam's reply when Sir Henry Clinton sent a messenger under a flag of truce to intercede for one such prisoner:

> Sir,—
>
> Edmund Palmer, an officer in the enemy's service, was taken as a spy, lurking within our lines. He has been tried as a spy, condemned as a spy, and shall be executed as a spy; and the flag is ordered to depart immediately.
>
> Israel Putnam
>
> P.S. He has been accordingly executed.

Meanwhile, disregarding the peril, David was building his new mine. In many ways it was similar to the powder magazine of the *Turtle*. However, the firing mechanism was not to be set off by clockwork. Instead, a series of wheels were to be provided, the largest one six inches in diameter, protruding an inch beyond the sides of the mine and equipped with spokes tipped with sharp iron points. If one of these mines were hauled aboard ship by a curious sailor, the iron points would catch on the ship's side, turn the wheels, and the wheels would then trip the gunlock, firing the powder.

By April David had the new device working properly, and on the twenty-second he appeared before Governor Trumbull and the Council of Safety, then in session at Lebanon, Connecticut. According to the official minutes, he exhibited "a specimen of a new invention for annoying ships." Immensely impressed by the demonstration, the Governor and Council gave him an order on "officers, agents and commissaries to afford him assistance of men, boats, powder, lead."

No doubt this was sincerely intended as a generous gesture, but there were many other drains upon the resources of Connecticut, and the assistance of men, boats, powder and lead could not be furnished if they did not exist. During the Revolution this one small state fitted out nearly 350 armed vessels; it is scarcely surprising if little aid was left over for the startling innovations David Bushnell proposed. However, for the next two years David considered himself to be working under a commission from the state, a commission to wage underwater warfare against the enemy whenever and wherever he could.

A few days after David appeared at Lebanon, the British brought the war right into Connecticut. Landing on the coast near the mouth of the Saugatuck River, a detachment of two thousand men under the infamous Governor Tryon marched toward Danbury, intent on destroying a large quantity of military supplies stored there. Early on Saturday afternoon, April 26, the enemy entered the town and began pillaging and plundering.

One old man, determined to save a bolt of cloth, tried to escape with it on horseback. Three light horsemen of the British troops galloped hard after him, shouting, "We'll have you yet, old daddy! We'll have you!"

"Not yet!" their quarry roared back.

The horsemen were almost upon him and were about to cut him down when the bolt of cloth began to unroll, fluttering out behind him like a streamer. The troopers' horses shied away, and the old man managed to escape.

As the vanguard of the British troops marched into town, several patriots fired upon them. The horsemen dashed up, cut the men down, and threw their bodies into a house, which they set on fire.

The troopers broke into the Episcopal church, which was filled to the galleries with three thousand barrels of pork and a thousand barrels of flour. These were rolled out and set on fire, turning the street, it was said, into a stream of boiling fat.

The next morning the marauding British celebrated the Sabbath by setting fire to nineteen houses, twenty-two stores and barns, and the meeting house of the New Danbury Society. In addition to the pork and flour, they destroyed several hundred barrels of beef, sixteen hundred tents, two thousand bushels of grain, as well as rice, army carriages and other supplies desperately needed by the Continental forces. This done, the redcoats marched away, having behaved with such barbarity that Sir William Howe disclaimed any connection with the raid.

When news of this pillage reached David, he used greater vigilance than ever. Once the British got word of what he was up to, they might swoop down at any moment. And he had little doubt that his life would be forfeit.

In a few months the British fleet was on the move again. "Black Dick" Howe dispatched a squadron under Sir Peter Parker to the waters around Rhode Island. The rest of the fleet sailed out of New York Bay, headed, it developed, for the Chesapeake to spearhead an attack upon Philadelphia, where the Continental Congress was in session.

From Saybrook David was in no position at this point to follow the fleet to Chesapeake Bay, but the squadron off Rhode Island offered fair game, if he could get close enough.

As it turned out, one of the ships came to him. In August the frigate *Cerberus,* commanded by Commodore John Symons, dropped anchor in Black Point Bay, a sheltered cove between Saybrook and New London. This was the very *Cerberus* that, several years before, had brought Sir William Howe, Sir Henry Clinton, and General John Burgoyne to Boston.

By Wednesday evening, August 13, David Bushnell had two mines in readiness for an attack. Each of the mines was composed of two boat-like vessels, twenty inches long and a foot wide, joined together by two four-foot iron bars, one at each end. Midway between the bars was an iron tube like a gun-barrel. The upper vessel protruded a few inches above the water, and the lower one, which was hidden beneath the water, was heavily ballasted and covered with lead. It was this lower vessel that contained the powder. The iron-spoked wheels, of course, served to trigger the firing mechanism.

These two floating mines were connected by a line about six hundred yards long, buoyed up by little sticks of wood at fixed distances.

With a whaleboat and some oarsmen, David set off from shore soon after darkness fell. When they got close to the *Cerberus,* they dropped one of the mines overboard.

Then, allowing the line to trail behind the boat, they rowed a considerable distance ahead of the ship until the entire length of the line had been played out. At this point they dropped the other mine in the water. The mines would float toward the ship, and the line connecting them would "swifter" the vessel, that is, encircle the hull lengthwise.

About eleven o'clock that night the crew of the *Cerberus* noticed a line towing astern. Believing someone had used it to veer away from the ship, Commodore Symons ordered the line to be hauled in. About 140 yards of rope was pulled aboard before the sailors were distracted by an uproar astern.

Lying astern of the *Cerberus* was a schooner, hidden from David's view when the mines were planted. The sailors aboard the schooner had spotted the other end of the line which Commodore Symons had seen. One of the men, taking it for a fishing line, began hauling it in. He had pulled in about thirty yards when he came upon the mine.

As the machine weighed more than a hundred pounds, he called upon some of his comrades for assistance. Together, they got it on deck. One of the seamen, formerly an ironmonger, was curious about the queer contraption and began moving a wheel backward and forward.

His curiosity proved fatal. Five minutes later the mine went off like a shot from a gun. The boat was demolished and the debris left in flames. The three men standing in the stern were killed immediately, and the fourth, standing forward, was blown into the water.

Commodore Symons immediately dispatched a boat to rescue the survivor and, after questioning him, ordered an inspection of the *Cerberus*. On the larboard side the sailors discovered the part of the line with the other mine. Symons snapped out an order that the line be cut at once, and the mine drifted away to an unrecorded fate. Then he rushed back to his cabin to draft a report of the incident for Rear Admiral Sir Peter Parker.

"As the ingenuity of these people is singular in their secret modes of mischief," he wrote, "and as I presume this is their first essay, I have thought it indispensably my duty to return and give you the earliest information of the circumstances, to prevent the like fatal accident happening to any of the advanced ships that may possibly be swiftered in the same manner, and to forbid all seamen from attempting hauling the line, or bringing the vessel near the ship, as it is filled with that kind of combustible that burns through in the water."

Symons was so intrigued by the mine that he had a model built, based on the description given by the survivor from the schooner.

This David Bushnell did not know at the time, nor did he know of the postscript to Commodore Symons' report: "It is therefore very fortunate I ordered the other to be cut away, for there is no knowing what damage it might have done, either to the ship or to the people."

"There is no knowing what damage it might have done" . . . once again luck had been against David. His invention had performed exactly as intended, and only by accident had it fallen in with the wrong target. But that target, though only a schooner, had been pulverized. Although this attack, like the ones by the *Turtle*, did not succeed from a tactical point of view, it did succeed strategically in spreading alarm among the British Navy. Many an officer and sailor slept uneasily after Commodore Symons' report had circulated. And their awareness of danger from these infernal machines undoubtedly deterred them from executing many coastal operations they might otherwise have attempted. Jonathan Trumbull later reported to Washington that the explosion had made the British "very cautious in their approaches to any of the neighboring shores." The destruction of the schooner and its crew were evidence that these were not the devices of an idle dreamer: they had a horrifying potential. In the war of nerves David Bushnell's attacks were achieving a signal victory.

X ➤ The Battle of the Kegs

FROM THE attack on the *Cerberus* David had learned several ways to make his mine more effective. When triggered by the spoked wheels, it could not be fired until hauled aboard ship, a method that left too much to chance. A mine was needed that would explode at the moment of contact, and David settled down to work on a new design.

Meanwhile, the British were busy. Down in Pennsylvania General Billy Howe took Philadelphia by storm. Fortunately for the Americans, this victory was offset by the surrender of "Gentleman Johnny" Burgoyne at Saratoga.

Aware that the British garrison in New York had been depleted, the Americans decided to make an attempt to recapture the strategic town. Among the forces that began moving down the east bank of the Hudson toward King's Bridge was Samuel Parsons' brigade. Like most of the patriot units, it was woefully ill-equipped. Parsons sent a plea for help to Governor Trumbull.

"In this station light horsemen are exceedingly wanted," he wrote. "I have at present four with me, which puts it beyond my power to effectually harass the enemy and answer other valuable purposes as the interest and safety of the country requires. I would therefore beg your Excellency to order me ten or twelve of the light horse of the State, which is the least number any person acquainted with this post will think necessary."

Tersely he added that even more basic equipment was needed: "Cloathing for the troops is now much wanted, especially shoes, stockings, and breeches, and will be very soon much more wanted."

And he had still another important request. "If Mr. Bushnell's projection for destroying the shipping can ever be of any use," Parsons wrote, "it can't be improved at any time to greater advantage than the present, nor at any place more likely to succeed than at this post."

By this time David Bushnell was busy elsewhere. He had been summoned to teach the British fleet at Philadelphia a lesson.

Defeated at the Battle of Germantown, Washington had retreated to a deep hollow scooped out from a low, rugged mountain in the west bank of the Schuylkill River, twenty-odd miles from Philadelphia. Here, clustered around the site of an old forge, were a few dwellings, and here, at Valley Forge, Washington took up winter quarters. The troops of Sir William Howe reveled in Philadelphia, and the ships of Admiral Lord Richard Howe cruised blithely up and down the Delaware.

To David, this situation offered a choice target, and he was delighted to answer a call for help from Bordentown, New Jersey, where Colonel Joseph Borden and a circle of ardent Whigs had heard of the exploits of the *Turtle*.

Bordentown is situated at the spot where the Delaware River bends like an elbow, seven miles below Trenton and twenty-six miles above Philadelphia. Lying on the crown of a hill, it commands a splendid view of the Delaware and the surrounding countryside. In the fall of 1777, when David journeyed there, the village was being used as a depot to store military supplies.

With the British so close, Colonel Borden and his friends feared that the presence of military stores would draw an attack by enemy troops. Many a night they sat late in the parlor of Colonel Borden's handsome house, concocting various projects that might annoy the redcoats and drive them from the river.

When Bushnell arrived, they offered generous assistance. Joseph Plowman, a mechanic, was charged with supervising construction of the mines, which were to incorporate several improvements upon those used in the attack on the *Cerberus*. When loaded with powder, they would explode immediately on rubbing against any object. This was accomplished by means of a springlock which would act as a detonator.

The springlocks were made by Robert Jackaway, who had a gunshop at the corner of Crosswicks Road and Main Street. Two brothers named Bunting, whose shop was across the street from Colonel Borden's home, did the blacksmithing, and the mines themselves were made in Colonel Borden's own cooper shop.

The new mines were to be fastened together in pairs by a connecting rope, much as those used on the *Cerberus* had been. However, this time the mines themselves were to be suspended from buoys. The buoys, which strongly resembled kegs, would be visible on the surface, and the mines would float beneath the waves. Once the mines had been carried downriver by the tide, it was hoped that the connecting rope would catch against the bow of a vessel, and that the mines would jostle against her sides and explode.

Keeping a watchful eye on the project was the man behind whose home the mines and keg-like buoys were being built. This was Francis Hopkinson, Colonel Borden's son-in-law and a member of the Continental Congress. A signer of the Declaration of Independence and often credited with designing the Stars and Stripes, he was one of the most versatile men of his time: a poet, a composer, later to become the designer of the Seal of the United States. In Congress he was chairman of the Continental Navy Board.

On behalf of the Navy Board Hopkinson wrote to Washington at Valley Forge on December 17, 1777: "I have the Pleasure of assuring you that everything goes on with Secrecy and Dispatch, to the Satisfaction of the Artist. We expect he will be enabled in a day or two to try the important Experiment."

The experiment was an attack by David's kegs on the British shipping at Philadelphia. All the ships lay out in the channel, moored in a long line that stretched the whole length of the waterfront.

On a cold night a few days after Christmas, David and a friend of Colonel Borden's named Carman made ready to set out on the mission. The kegs and mines were loaded in a whaleboat, which set off from the foot of Market Street. More than twenty of the kegs had been prepared, and it was a perilous venture to attempt to pilot them down the Delaware.

"I was unacquainted with the river," David later wrote, "and obliged to depend upon a gentleman very imperfectly acquainted with that part of it, as I afterwards found."

The whaleboat moved as close to the British shipping as Carman dared go. It was an extremely dark night, overcast by storm clouds, with little moonlight. Both David and Carman, deceived by the darkness, believed themselves to be within a thousand feet of the shipping. Actually, they were nowhere near so close.

Relieved to be rid of their explosive cargo, David and Carman set the kegs and mines loose. They were supposed to drift down with the ebbing tide upon the British shipping below. But the two men had miscalculated the distance, and they had also miscalculated the swiftness of the tides. Moreover, the river had become clogged with floating ice. The passage of the kegs toward their target was delayed, and instead of being held together in a mass, they became scattered.

Another unfortunate result of the delay was that a few of the targets departed before the kegs arrived. Some of the British fleet cleared from the Delaware on December 29; by January 2 they had anchored safely at Rhode Island.

A number of the ships left at Philadelphia also were taken out of harm's way. Fearing the ice that was forming over the river, the British warped in their vessels to the wharves.

One pair of kegs and mines arrived earlier than the rest, floating in the river opposite to the city. Two boys saw the strange buoys. Their curiosity aroused, they jumped into a small boat and rowed out to investigate. When they attempted to pull one of the kegs into the boat, the device burst with a great explosion and, as a newspaper reported, "blew up the unfortunate boys." This occurred some distance from the British sentinels, and no general alarm was raised.

Finally, about dawn on Monday, January 5, the rest of the floating mines reached the city. The crew of a barge pulled one of the kegs aboard. When it was detonated, four of the hands were killed and the rest severely wounded. This time an alarm spread throughout the entire city, throwing everyone into confusion. Men, women and children barricaded themselves in their homes. British troops ran to the assigned places of muster. Drums and trumpets sounded, and the cavalry dashed up and down the street in an uproar. Before long the wharves and the decks of all the ships in port were lined with spectators. Dozens of rumors flew about, and everyone had a different opinion of what the kegs represented.

Some said the kegs were filled with armed rebels; they swore they had seen bayonets sticking out of the bungholes of the kegs. The rebels would come forth in the dead of night, as the

Greeks did from the Trojan Horse, and take the city by surprise.

Others said that the kegs were the products of a fiendish magician, that they had the power to clamber up over the wharves at night and go rolling through the city streets, bursting into flames and destroying everything in their path.

Still others came closer to the truth. The kegs, they said, "were charged with the most inveterate combustibles, to be kindled by secret machinery, and setting the whole Delaware in flames, were to consume all the shipping in the harbor."

The battle that followed was gleefully reported by a "correspondent" in the *New Jersey Gazette* a few weeks later. Evidence indicates that the anonymous writer was none other than Francis Hopkinson:

". . . it was surprising to behold the incessant blaze that was kept up against the enemy, the kegs.

"Both officers and men exhibited the most unparalleled skill and bravery on the occasion . . . From the *Roebuck* and other ships of war, whole broadsides were poured into the Delaware. In short, not a wandering ship, stick, or drift-log, but felt the vigour of the British arms.

"The action began about sunrise, and would have been compleated with great success by noon, had not an old market woman coming down the river with provisions, unfortunately let a small keg of butter fall over-board, which (as it was then ebb) floated down to the scene of the action. At the sight of this unexpected reinforcement of the enemy, the battle was renewed with fresh fury—the firing was incessant till the evening closed the affair. The kegs were either totally demolished or obliged to fly, as none of them have shown their *heads* since. It is said his Excellency, Lord Howe, has dispatched a swift sailing packet with an account of this victory, to the court of London. In a word, Monday the 5th of January

1778, must ever be distinguished in history for the memorable
BATTLE OF THE KEGS."

Francis Hopkinson soon made sure that the British would
not forget the attempt. Within a few weeks he had composed
a rousing ballad called, appropriately, "British Valour Displayed: Or, The Battle of the Kegs." From the moment it was
first published in the *Pennsylvania Packet*, it became a great
hit among the Continental troops. For the soldiers who sang
the verses around the campfires at Valley Forge, it was one of
the few bright spots of the miserable winter, and it remained a
favorite for years to come.

But even without Hopkinson's ballad, the British were unlikely to forget the Battle of the Kegs. The panic and alarm
on the ships and in the streets of Philadelphia had been no
laughing matter. And once again the British had proof that
this new weapon could be lethal: a rowboat and a barge had
been demolished. The next time it might well be a man-of-war.

The British still held the preponderance of sea power, but
their confidence in the invincibility of the navy had received
a severe blow. As long as they remained at Philadelphia every
piece of flotsam that appeared was viewed with apprehension,
and orders were issued that any floating object that could not
be identified was to be fired upon.

With the attack on the *Cerberus* and the attack on the shipping at Philadelphia, David Bushnell had not achieved spec-
tacular results, but he had proved his point: warfare could be
waged with floating mines. The next attack—or the one after
that—might help to turn the tide of the war. One dramatic
success, and he was convinced that support would be forthcoming to build a fleet of floating mines.

XI ➤ The British
Capture a Prize

WHEN DAVID returned to Saybrook in the spring of 1778, his hopes and spirits were high. He seemed to be on the brink of success in his attempts to serve his country with his devices for submarine warfare.

But he had no money, and no prospects of money. He could always find a home with Ezra, but Ezra now had been married for more than a year to young Patience Lord. David could not ask him to contribute toward the building of mines.

In early April he again went before Governor Trumbull and the Council to beg for assistance. The state treasury was depleted, so Trumbull, always his supporter, agreed to request the Connecticut delegates in Congress to see if aid could be obtained from Congress itself.

With surprising speed, the delegates replied on April 29, requesting an account of David's expenses. "We are fully of the opinion," they wrote, "that his genious ought to be encouraged and Rewarded at a Continental Expence, and shall take the Earliest Opportunity to urge it."

"His genious"—more and more it was being recognized.

While he was waiting for funds with which to construct new mines, David took time to obtain a Master's degree from Yale.

He was not a man content to be idle.

College president Ezra Stiles noted in his diary on September 9 that he had conferred degrees upon forty-two Masters. "I threw up my fee," he wrote, "& referred myself to the Liberality of the Graduates for this Commencement." Then he added, "Only this to be no precedent for the future." It seems that out of the forty-two candidates, eleven—including David Bushnell—paid him nothing at all.

Meanwhile, the war, dormant for many months, had erupted into activity. The French made an alliance with the United States and went to war against the British. Cold, haughty Sir Henry Clinton replaced genial William Howe as commander of the British forces and began moving them from Philadelphia toward New York. Pulling the Americans out of their encampment at Valley Forge, Washington followed, to grapple with the enemy at Monmouth. The battle was indecisive. The British went on to fortify themselves in New York, and Washington moved to White Plains. Once again the Revolution settled down to a series of scattered skirmishes. The monotony was broken only twice—by the arrival of the French fleet in July and by an abortive Franco-American attack on Newport in August. One outcome of this battle undoubtedly gave David great pleasure: to keep the *Cerberus* from falling into French hands, the British themselves set her on fire.

By early 1779 Connecticut was being threatened with invasion. Samuel Parsons, stationed with his troops at Lyme, was worried about the defenses of New London, only fifteen miles away. Rumors had been flying that a huge British fleet was on the way. At sunset on March 23 the frigate *Renown* appeared at the mouth of the Thames River at New London and dropped anchor. The townspeople thought the attack would come at any moment.

"On the whole," Parsons wrote to Governor Trumbull the

next day, "we are in a state which affords me very little hope of preventing the enemy from destroying the town. I have sent for Bushnell to see if we can dislodge the ship which is now said to block up the harbor."

David, in his solitary way, was continuing to harass the British. But with his reticence and his passion for secrecy, he left no account of exactly what he attempted and how well he succeeded during this period. Obviously, his high hopes after the Battle of the Kegs were not being realized, or his contemporaries would have noted his triumphs.

And a few weeks later his guerrilla activities were brought to a halt in a dramatic manner.

At this time Connecticut was being harried by a number of small-boat expeditions, manned by marauding, plundering Tories encouraged by the British. Late on May 1 nine of these Tories set out in a whaleboat from Lloyd's Neck, a headland between Oyster Bay and Huntington on Long Island. Their boat, about thirty feet in length, was sharp and light, built for speed and silence.

On this dark, moonless night they headed for Fairfield on the Connecticut shore. Their quarry was General Gold S. Silliman, charged with defending that portion of the coast. Among the marauders was a carpenter who had once been employed by Silliman and knew his way about the grounds and house. Leaving one man to guard the boat, the remaining eight Tories crept up to the house about midnight, broke in, seized Silliman and his son, and carried them back to the boat. After crossing the Sound, the two prisoners were turned over to the British.

On May 6 the marauders were out again. This time a party landed at Middlesex, near Norwalk, seeking to kidnap a Captain Selleck. When they discovered their quarry had eluded them, they decided to carry away three of the inhabitants of the neighborhood and a fourth man as well, a stranger to the other three captives, a man of about forty years, quiet, unassuming, and, they thought, of little significance. But they did not want to return to Long Island empty-handed.

The marauders had done better than they knew. The next day Israel Putnam dashed off a letter to General Washington. "I am unhappy to inform your Excellency that . . . the ingenious Dr. Bushnell fell into their hands." David, Putnam reported, "was there in the prosecution of his unremitting endeavors to destroy the enemy's shipping."

By good fortune, Putnam added, as Bushnell "is personally known to very few people, it is possible that he may not be discovered by his real name or character, and may be considered of less consequence than he actually is."

David Bushnell was carried off to New York as a prisoner. One story (without much foundation in fact) says that aboard a prison ship he acted the part of the village idiot. One day an officer discovered him hacking away at the rigging with a hatchet. Asked what he was doing, David replied that in the spring he always cut away the brush and cleared up the land. The officer reported the incident to the commander of the frigate, and the commander ordered the "fool" put ashore. Once David was safe and sound, so the story says, he sent off a note informing the commander of the prison ship who he was.

Actually, Bushnell's situation was extremely perilous. British prison ships were places of horrible cruelty and suffering. Prisoners were allowed on deck only after sunset, and then one at a time. All the rest of the day and night they lay crowded in the hold, where, as one soldier reported, "the steam was enough to scald the skin and take away the Breath—the stench enough to poison the air all around."

The prisons on land were equally shocking. Joshua Loring, the commissary of prisoners, was so loathsome that his cruelty to prisoners was compared to the conduct of barbaric Turks.

Israel Putnam hurried to secure David's release before the British learned they held the man whose floating mines posed such a threat. Immediately after writing to Washington, Putnam dashed off a letter to Governor Trumbull, proposing that some of the British prisoners held in the Hartford gaol be exchanged for David and several other Americans. He wished it to be a routine exchange, so that the British would not be alerted to the true value of David Bushnell.

On May 13 the Governor and Council resolved that nine British prisoners be delivered into the hands of Brigadier General Parsons, to be sent by him into New York in exchange for nine Americans, including David.

The notorious Joshua Loring agreed to the exchange, and the Americans were turned over to General Parsons. David was fortunate. Many Americans held by the British languished in prison for years—if they managed to cling to life that long.

No letters in which David described his ordeal while imprisoned at New York have ever come to light. However, it is evident that it was a turning point in his life. While in prison he decided to abandon his attempts at guerrilla warfare, to act no more as a one-man task force, to give up his struggle to scrape together funds to build his mines. He was through acting as a free agent. He would find some other way to serve his country.

Within little more than a week after his exchange he presented himself to Governor Trumbull to request a favor. He had heard that Washington was attempting to form a Corps of Sappers and Miners to aid the Corps of Engineers, in which most of the officers were highly skilled Frenchmen. In the Sappers and Miners, David thought, might lie the opportunity he sought. Within the army, with its support, he might be able, perhaps, to rebuild the *Turtle*, he might have occasion to use his mines as part of the military tactics in a campaign, he might even see a way to devise some new weapon that could be brought to bear on the enemy.

Trumbull was happy to oblige. "I suppose your Excellency is not wholly unacquainted with the character of Mr. David Bushnell, the bearer," he wrote. "His inventions for annoying the enemy's shipping are new and ingenious . . . . The vigilance practised in guarding the shipping has, I suppose, been the only means of preventing such execution as would have been attended with very alarming and beneficial consequences. He has, with persevering and indefatigable industry, pursued the object with very little prospect of any other reward than that of serving his country. . . ."

Trumbull proposed that David be appointed to a captaincy in the Corps of Sappers and Miners. "It is a pity," he stated, "that so promising a genius should not be encouraged. . . . From his abilities, genius, and integrity, I should judge him capable to execute [his duties] with honor and advantage."

The Council, Trumbull added, joined with him in the recommendation.

And with the highest hopes, David set out for Washington's headquarters.

XII ➤ The Sappers and Miners

ARMED WITH his fine endorsement from Governor Trumbull, David presented himself to General Washington. He encountered no difficulties. The Corps of Sappers and Miners was not an especially popular outfit, and qualified applicants were hard to come by.

Although Washington had called for officers to take commissions in the corps more than a year earlier, it was not properly organized until the summer of 1779, just about the time David appeared in camp, and even then it was far from full strength.

For one thing, the corps had been placed under the command of Brigadier General Louis le Bèque de Presle Du Portail, chevalier of France, who, like the Marquis de Lafayette, had thrown in his lot with the American cause. Long since, as commander of the Corps of Engineers, he had shown he knew how to get a job done. But he was haughty, opinionated, and an unrelenting taskmaster—qualities which did not endear him to his men.

For another thing, it was plain from the start that the Sappers and Miners were to encounter hard work, great danger, and little glory. "On a march, in the vicinity of the enemy," ran the orders, "a detachment of the Companies of Sappers and Miners shall be stationed at the head of the column, directly after the Van Guard for the purpose of opening and mending the roads and removing obstructions." In addition, Congress decreed that they were "to repair injuries done to the works by the enemy's fire, and to prosecute works in the face of it." This was no deterrent to David. He had no fear of danger, and he positively thrived on hard work. It suited him better than ease.

Of the officers, a knowledge of practical geometry and drawing was required. The enlisted men were to be able to write a good hand—and have strong backs. They would learn how to construct field works of every kind—to dig the narrow trenches called saps, dispose of the earth, cut the slopes, face the works with turf or sod, cut and fix palisades, and build any other kind of work necessary for the attack or defense of positions. In addition, when preparing for a siege, they would have to make fascines and gabions. The former were sticks tied in bundles and used to strengthen ramparts; the latter were basket-like contrivances to be filled with earth in constructing breastworks. It was tedious and tiresome work.

No one was surprised that applicants for the corps were not numerous. Washington promised extra pay in case of extraordinary fatigue or danger, but from bitter experience every soldier in the Continental Army knew that pay was slow in coming, if it came at all. But David was well accustomed to the lack of money.

On August 2, 1779, less than a month before his thirty-ninth birthday, David Bushnell was one of three captain lieutenants appointed after a rigorous examination by Brigadier General Du Portail. At the same time, three captains and two first lieutenants were appointed, and three companies of Sappers and Miners were formally organized. Some of the officers were immediately sent out to recruit more men.

Together with the main body of the army, the handful of

men in the Sappers and Miners went into winter quarters at Jockey Hollow, a spot about three miles southwest of Morristown, New Jersey. For the Continental troops, the future seemed grimmer than ever. The British had captured Savannah, and rumors were flying that Sir Henry Clinton was about to sail from New York to attack Charleston.

David had faced hardships before, but none had been so terrible as those of that winter, an ordeal much worse, many said, than the horrors of the previous winter at Valley Forge. It took weeks to complete the log huts. The few officers and men lucky enough to have tents found they offered slight protection against the cold winter winds that ripped through the encampment. Some of the soldiers were half-naked, without blankets, coats or shoes. "Our only food is miserable fresh beef, without bread, salt, or vegetables," wrote one of the officers, and on some days there was not even the miserable fresh beef. The day before Christmas brought a slight consolation: orders directed that the Sappers and Miners be furnished with shirts and linen.

The men were grumbling about other things than cold and hunger. The Continental paper money was depreciating alarmingly, and if the soldiers were paid at all, the pay was paper, with no allowance for depreciation. It was said that with four months' pay a private could scarcely buy a bushel of wheat for his family, that a colonel's pay would not purchase oats for his horse.

At dusk one evening toward the end of May, the discontent came to a head. Two regiments of Parsons' Connecticut troops assembled and declared they were going to march home bag and baggage. Other troops were called out to restore order, and it took some persuasive talking on the part of the officers to get the miserable, half-starving men to return to their huts.

Spies carried news of the near-mutiny to the British, and soon handbills printed by the enemy were being passed around camp, urging the soldiers to desert. Then, in June, believing that the Continental troops were ready to throw up their arms, the British came swarming over from Staten Island to invade New Jersey. The Americans stood firm.

By July the Sappers and Miners were better off, barracked in the old meetinghouse at Peekskill, a small village below West Point on the opposite bank of the Hudson. Their ranks now were increased by a forced draft from among the various regiments, and they took pride in their new official uniform: a blue coat with buff facings, red linings, buff underclothes and the epaulettes of their respective ranks.

In the months that followed Captain Lieutenant Bushnell's movements are obscured, almost as if he had been swallowed up by the anonymity of the military machine. On September 20 Governor Trumbull and the Connecticut Council of Safety granted him £20 for an unspecified purpose, at a time when the treasury was low, with many other demands upon it. No record survives to indicate how the money was used.

The Sappers and Miners had now moved down from Peekskill to Dobbs' Ferry, where, near the ferry itself, they built a blockhouse and set up a battery to fire upon any British shipping that ventured past.

A few days before they actually got the battery in place, the British sloop-of-war *Vulture* had moved up the river and dropped anchor off Teller's Point, about midway between Dobbs' Ferry and West Point. No one, however, had any fears about the safety of West Point. Benedict Arnold had just been placed in command of the fort, and Arnold had long since proved himself a superb general. He had, of course, been in trouble recently over his financial affairs; he had even faced a court-martial and been reprimanded by Washington. But that, the soldiers thought, had nothing to do with his brilliance and courage in the field.

As it turned out, the *Vulture* had swooped up the river at Arnold's invitation. He had made plans to turn over the fort to the enemy. On the night of September 21, Major John André, the young, handsome adjutant-general of the British Army, was aboard the *Vulture*. Shortly before midnight, wearing a blue greatcoat over his uniform, he boarded a rowboat that crossed to the west bank of the river and landed him at a solitary spot at the foot of a mountain called the Long Clove. There, hidden among the thickets, was General Benedict Arnold.

Arnold had come with the plans of the defenses of West Point; André with authority to settle the terms of payment. Until dawn the two conspirators talked. With daylight they concealed themselves in the nearby home of Joshua Hett Smith (who later claimed ignorance of their plot).

Meanwhile, to André's dismay, the Americans cannonaded the *Vuture;* cutting her cables, she moved down the river. André, forced to return to British headquarters in New York by land, decided to exchange his military coat for a civilian coat of Smith's. The decision was fatal. On the way to New York he was seized, his papers discovered, and he was arrested as a spy.

Arnold's treachery was not yet suspected. When the messenger arrived with news of André's capture, Arnold mounted his messenger's horse, galloped down to a landing place where his six-oared barge was moored, and ordered his men to row with all haste for the *Vulture*. Not realizing what was afoot, the men obeyed, and when the *Vulture* was reached Arnold turned them over to the British as prisoners.

That evening the *Vulture* moved down the Hudson toward New York. Unaware that Arnold was aboard—or even that he was a traitor—the Sappers and Miners fired at her as she passed the battery at Dobbs' Ferry. The cannon fire was ineffectual, and the sloop moved on undamaged.

A week later at Tappan, a hamlet across the Hudson from Dobbs' Ferry, Major John André was hanged, after a court-martial. Along with other Continental troops, a good many of the Sappers and Miners witnessed the execution, and perhaps David Bushnell was among them. He must have thought back to Nathan Hale, hanged by the British four years before without benefit of trial. Whereas André's fate attracted widespread attention (Sir Henry Clinton made frantic attempts to save him)—and considerable pity even among his captors —Hale had died before his compatriots even knew of his capture, and his death was almost unnoticed by the public.

And David was puzzled by the shocking revelations about Benedict Arnold. This man, denounced as a traitor of the blackest dye, was the same man who had been such a hero to David and all the boys at Yale back in 1775 when he defied the town fathers and seized the ammunition before marching off to Boston! The American forces had already known deserters, even a few traitors, but none before had been despised so heartily.

Strengthening the fortifications at West Point was now imperative. Major General Nathanael Greene was temporarily placed in command of the post and ordered to march there immediately with sizable reinforcements, including the Corps of Sappers and Miners. Moving up to Peekskill, Captain Lieutenant Bushnell and the other officers and men obtained flat-bottomed boats to carry themselves and their baggage the rest of the way up the river to West Point. The redoubts and batteries had been built on a natural platform of rocks, rising more than 150 feet above the waters of the Hudson and overlooking the country for thirty miles around.

Because the only barracks available were ramshackle, they set about building new ones. For the timber they had to go about six miles downriver to fell trees, then carry the logs to the river's edge, where the rafts were waiting to transport them upstream. Not until New Year's Day were the barracks ready for the officers and men to move in.

It was dull, unimaginative work, and David was beginning to doubt the wisdom of having joined the corps. The opportunity for initiative was slight, and the chance to exercise mechanical genius was non-existent. When, he often wondered, would he be able to put his submarine devices to work again? But as the weeks lengthened into months, and the months into years, he began to fit in.

During this period Benedict Arnold, lately appointed a brigadier general in His Majesty's service, had been pillaging Virginia. Now he entrenched himself and his troops at Portsmouth, opposite Norfolk. Late in February, 1781, the Sappers and Miners were part of a detachment of twelve hundred men dispatched under the ardent young Marquis de Lafayette to capture Arnold.

"You are to do no act whatever," ran Lafayette's orders, "that directly or by implication may screen him from the punishment due to his treason and desertion, which, if he should fall into your hands, you will execute in the most summary manner."

Here, at last, David thought, would be a chance for action. But the attempt failed, and the Miners, who had got as far as Annapolis, were back at West Point by April.

As an officer, David was more popular with his superiors than with his subordinates. With his passion for secrecy, he never talked to the men about the attack on the *Eagle*; he never mentioned the part he had played in "The Battle of the Kegs." All the troops saw was a man approaching forty, not in the best of health, taciturn, slightly embittered, and as much of a martinet as Du Portail about adhering to duty and doing a job well.

Yet David always had the best interests of his men at heart. When he learned that the Council of Safety at Hartford was adjusting the pay of the troops in the Connecticut line to make up for the depreciation of the Continental paper money, he petitioned that the same allowances be made for the men from Connecticut in the Sappers and Miners. Also signing the petition were his superior officer, Captain James Beebe (of whom Alexander Hamilton had written, "He sings well and that's all"), and Captain Lieutenant Moses Cleaveland (later to found Cleveland, Ohio). The petition—the first of several Captain Lieutenant Bushnell made on behalf of the troops—was granted.

He and the others in his company soon had a good reason to celebrate. Since entering the corps they had not received a penny of pay. Now, in one lump payment, David received his pay and subsistence from August, 1779, through March, 1780, "it being one thousand Eighteen dollars and one third—£305.0.0." A few days later he received his April, 1780, pay: $133⅓. More than a year's pay still was due, but he was faring no worse than most of the soldiers, and better than some.

Then more good fortune befell him. On June 8 Captain Beebe resigned, and David was appointed captain. He was moving ahead, even if not in the direction he had intended.

Washington and the French allies now decided to lay siege to New York, in the hope either that the town would fall, or that Sir Henry Clinton would be forced to withdraw some of his forces from the South, where the Americans were hard pressed. The Sappers and Miners, together with the Engineers, were busily making preparations, constructing fascines and gabions, and taking part in the numerous movements to reconnoiter the enemy's positions. On one of these forays, Captain Bushnell had charge of a whaleboat to convey men down the Hudson toward King's Bridge. It was a sector that brought back somber memories to David, for near here the *Turtle* had been sunk.

While the troops were carrying out these movements, two items of intelligence reached Washington. He learned that his ally, Admiral de Grasse, was sailing from the West Indies with the French fleet, bound for Chesapeake Bay. And he learned that his enemy, Lord Cornwallis, had holed up with his troops near the lower end of the Chesapeake, at Yorktown, believing it an ideal naval base for communication with Sir Henry Clinton in New York.

Abruptly abandoning the projected siege of New York, Washington decided to move south with his troops, leaving only a token force to guard West Point. The new plan was kept so secret that most of the soldiers failed to realize their destination until well on the way.

The march was rapid. The Sappers and Miners passed through Jersey and on to Philadelphia, where the weather was warm and dry, and clouds of dust blinded their eyes and covered their bodies. Here they paused for a few days, to pack shells, shot and other military supplies, and to draw new clothing to replace a part of their tattered uniforms. Captain Bushnell had aroused the ire of some of the enlisted men by his unswerving insistence on rigid discipline, and on the march out of Philadelphia they took revenge by sneaking up and—before he could spot the culprits—dumping him off a rail fence into a ditch.

At what is now Elkton, Maryland, a fleet of about eighty vessels was waiting to transport the troops down the Chesapeake. By September 26 they had reached Yorktown, encamping in a large wood about a mile and a half from the enemy's line of redoubts. They were in a level country, a land of pine forests, holly and laurel.

Yorktown, with only about sixty buildings, was little more than a village, standing on a high bluff covered with sandy soil, on the south side of the York River about eleven miles from its mouth. For Cornwallis and his seven to eight thousand men, it might have been a fine naval base, but it offered few defenses against an attack by land. All Cornwallis could do was to rely on the water for protection on one side, and on the other side throw up a line of earthworks with about ten redoubts and fourteen batteries. Until reinforcements could arrive by sea from Sir Henry Clinton in New York, he hoped this would hold off the sixteen thousand or more besiegers who had formed a half-circle around the town.

The plan for the siege was this: While an incessant bombardment was kept up, a series of trenches would be constructed in parallel lines. Each line would be closer to the town than the one before. The first parallel was to be six to eight hundred feet from the enemy; earth would be shoveled up over the fascines to form parapets. From this parallel line, the narrow trenches called saps would be dug at angles, leading forward toward the enemy; these would be protected by the gabions constructed earlier. When the saps had been dug leading forward three hundred yards from the first parallel, then a second line of trenches would be dug parallel to the first. This process would be repeated until the trenches were close enough to the enemy for the infantry to attack.

The allied troops spent most of the first week in October preparing the fascines and gabions, bringing up the guns, and surveying the approaches. All the while the British kept up a furious cannonade. On October 2, for example, 351 shot were fired between sunrise and sunset.

The Miners and Engineers were sent out the night of October 5 to start work on the first parallel, but a fierce rainstorm drove them back. The following night Captain Bushnell and the other officers were out again, along with fatigue parties, moving with great silence and secrecy, carrying fascines and entrenching tools on their shoulders. Behind them were horses drawing cannon and wagons loaded with sandbags. Not until daylight did the British wake up to what was going on. Although they kept up an unceasing fire for three or four days, it did not prevent the allies from opening the second parallel on October 11 within three hundred yards of the British works.

This was more to David's taste. He and the others, step by step, trench by trench, were making visible progress toward the enemy. The corps had given him no opening to use his submarine mines, but here, at least, he was doing something active to help defeat the British.

Two of the enemy redoubts, Numbers 9 and 10, kept up such a steady fire that the allies could not extend the second parallel all the way to the river. Capture of the two forts was a necessity. The French were detailed to storm Redoubt Number 9; the Americans, Redoubt Number 10. The attack was set for the night of October 14.

Commanding the Americans was Lieutenant Colonel Alexander Hamilton. Lafayette had wished to place a French officer in charge, with the result that Hamilton took his case direct to Washington himself, who settled the matter in Hamilton's favor. With Hamilton went some of the Sappers and Miners under Captain James Gilliland and Captain Lieutenant David Kirkpatrick. Those Sappers and Miners left in the rear were commanded by Captain Bushnell. Unlike Hamilton, who had grown close to Washington when his aide, David Bushnell could not go to the Commander-in-Chief to protest being left behind.

Close to eight o'clock, rockets were set off as a signal for the joint attack by the Americans and the French, and the two groups moved forward toward the redoubts.

Protecting each of the redoubts were obstacles known as abatis, formed of tree branches cut sharp as spikes and fixed in the ground, pointing outward toward the attackers. The Miners had been given axes and told to move in the van of the troops in order to cut through these abatis.

When the American soldiers started to move, however, they rushed ahead pell-mell without waiting for the Miners to go to work. They broke through the obstructions, scrambled through the ditch, scaled the parapet and captured the fort— all within ten minutes of starting out.

The Miners had rushed ahead with them. "Captain Gilliland with the detachment of sappers and miners," wrote Lieutenant Colonel Hamilton, "acquitted themselves in a manner that did them great honor." And David Kirkpatrick, he added, "received a wound in the ditch."

According to Hamilton's official report, the Continental losses in storming Redoubt Number 10 were nine killed and thirty-two wounded. The French, though also victorious in the attack on Redoubt Number 9, suffered nearly three times as many casualties. They had paused while the abatis were cut through.

By morning both the redoubts had been included in the second parallel, and the siege continued. Cornwallis, on the sixteenth, made two desperate attempts. Before daybreak he ordered an attack on two allied batteries, hoping to spike the guns; the attackers failed to accomplish their mission. After dark he tried to evacuate his troops to the opposite side of the river, hoping to escape; but at midnight a storm arose, and the parties were driven back.

"We at that time could not fire a single gun," reported

Cornwallis. "I therefore proposed to capitulate."

At ten o'clock the following morning Cornwallis sent forward an officer, waving a white handkerchief, to ask for the terms of surrender. Two days later, at two o'clock in the afternoon, the British marched out of Yorktown, dressed in splendid new uniforms, with colors cased and the bands playing "The World Turned Upside Down." Drawn up on the left were the French, brilliant in their white uniforms. On the right were the Americans, ragged and war-weary, but bursting with pride. Cornwallis could not face the humiliation of surrender; pleading illness, he sent out his sword by another officer.

The siege of Yorktown was over. And so, thought many of the exhausted Continentals, was the war.

David Bushnell was as thankful as the rest. Yet his submarine, his mines . . . they were no longer needed by the American cause. For the duration of his service he knew he must bend his thoughts and energies to be, simply, a good officer in the Corps of Sappers and Miners. The tide of events had swept the British Navy beyond his reach.

XIII ≻ "I Have Ever Wished
to Be Silent . . ."

THE SURRENDER at Yorktown aroused jubilation such as the country had never before seen. As the couriers rode hard, the tide of celebration spread north and west and south. On the village greens, before the town courthouses, in the city squares, crowds gathered, bonfires were lit, and salutes fired. And, in the churches, there was solemn thanksgiving.

The victory was unexpected, magnificent, complete. Like the soldiers in Virginia, people everywhere felt that the end of British power in America had come.

Yet the British still held Savannah, Charleston, Wilmington and New York. Peace might be on the way, but it was to be a long time in arriving.

While the exodus of the allied armies from Yorktown began, David Bushnell and a handful of the Sappers and Miners were given a duty which they considered highly distasteful after the excitement of combat. They were sent on board a small schooner with more than twenty tons of salted beef stored in its hold. Their task was to dole it out as rations to whatever troops had not yet departed. The men grew bored and restless, and the weather turned cold and stormy. After nearly three weeks most of the beef was gone, and David moved the small detachment posthaste up the Chesapeake, where they joined the rest of the corps on a march through Philadelphia to winter quarters at Burlington, New Jersey.

Their new barracks was by far the most elegant quarters they had seen: a handsome mansion, once the residence of the Royal Governor. This was the only taste of luxury they had, for they were still without adequate clothes, without money and sometimes without food. An outbreak of what seemed to be a species of yellow fever made them even more wretched.

By April they were back at Constitution Island, opposite West Point, blasting rocks to be used in repairing the works, or building a new barracks, large enough to quarter two or three regiments.

Soon David was again in touch with the Connecticut General Assembly about money, petitioning that the Connecticut members of the Miners might be paid on the same footing as soldiers in the Connecticut line. This petition was granted, but he was not always to be so successful.

Time was heavy on his hands, and his ways were more solitary than ever. Constitution Island was rugged and uneven, and the spot David picked for his tent was apart from those of the men, a desolate place in an old gravel pit. Here, at least, he could be by himself, away from the squabbles that constantly broke out among the men. They felt they were marking time, and they were itching to get back to their families and farms.

But what was David to return to? He had sold his farm, spent every penny he possessed on the *Turtle*, and bad luck had cursed every attempt he had made with the *Turtle* or with his floating mines. He was now forty-two, unmarried, bankrupt in purse and in spirit. And the future promised little.

He moved alone. Near the river bank on the island were

the ruins of an old barracks, the stones of the foundations still remaining. Around them bushes had grown up. Here, toward sunset whenever the weather was good, David used to go and pace up and down in the fading light, often close to despair.

Captain James Gilliland, who had led the corps in the attack on Redoubt Number 10 at Yorktown, resigned in October, 1782, and now David was usually the officer commanding the corps. It brought him little happiness.

One of his junior officers, Captain Lieutenant Peter Taulman, was brash and unruly. He had taken an unreasonable dislike to David and never missed a chance to flout him. Even worse, he encouraged another officer, Captain Lieutenant David Kirkpatrick (who had been wounded at Yorktown) to join his insubordination.

On December 31, for example, David as a matter of routine sent Taulman a form on which he was to make out a return for provisions for the troops in his company. Taulman deliberately neglected to fill out the form.

On New Year's Day matters came to a head. Without explanation Taulman and Kirkpatrick burst into Captain Bushnell's quarters in the barracks on Constitution Island. Behind them came soldiers carrying their baggage. Astounded by this impudence, David ordered the soldiers to take the baggage out, only to have the order countermanded by the insubordinate junior officers. Facing the two squarely, David now ordered them to have the baggage removed.

"Your order is not sufficient," Taulman said, openly defiant.

When Bushnell told him to consider himself under arrest, Taulman retired to the other side of the room. "I wish," he said to Kirkpatrick, "you would order those things in. Don't you see he has put me under arrest?"

"They are not my things," Kirkpatrick answered, but immediately ordered his own baggage in.

"I'll not consider myself under arrest till I receive it in writing," Taulman muttered and once again ordered the soldiers to bring in his baggage, even picking up several pieces himself. Encouraged by Taulman and Kirkpatrick, the soldiers disobeyed Captain Bushnell.

"Your order is not sufficient," Taulman repeated. "You are nobody. You are no gentleman."

The incident was approaching mutiny. Quickly Bushnell wrote out an order placing Taulman under arrest and handed it to him.

"You have nothing to do with me," Taulman raged. "I should think you would know more about duty than to give orders to an officer under arrest. *You* pretend to know more than I, who have been three years longer than you in service."

At this point Captain Bushnell went directly to Major General Knox, the garrison commander, to report the insubordination, and when he returned, Taulman, Kirkpatrick, the soldiers and the baggage still were in his quarters. Calling in two other officers, he repeated the orders to Taulman and Kirkpatrick and then placed them under guard.

Washington, outraged, ordered a General Court-martial. Taulman was sentenced to be reprimanded and suspended from service for three months; Kirkpatrick, to be reprimanded. The Commander-in-Chief issued a stinging rebuke, calling their behavior a "blot which now stains a page in the Records of the Army . . . an outrageous infraction of military Decipline."

But Captain Bushnell's troubles were not yet over. All of a sudden—no one ever found out why—a certain Captain Joseph de Lazen of the Corps of Engineers took it into his head to appear at West Point and announce that he was assuming command of the Sappers and Miners. Washington put a stop to this impertinence immediately, affirming that Captain Bushnell was properly the corps commander and ordering Captain de Lazen to present himself at headquarters to explain on whose authority he had acted.

Incidents of this sort were happening with more and more frequency throughout the army. The soldiers were restless and bored. Eighteen months had passed since the victory at Yorktown that had seemed to promise an end to the war. Finally, on April 19, 1783, it was announced to the troops that the provisional treaty of peace had been signed and ratified by Congress. By mid-June most of the soldiers had been granted furloughs and were on their way home; final discharges would be handed out when the formal peace treaty had been signed.

Captain Bushnell was one of the few who stayed on in the army after June. His signature appears on army returns from Newburgh and West Point and Constitution Island. In September he was granted forage for his horse, a privilege usually denied officers in the Sappers and Miners, and allowed to him only because he had been performing the duties of a staff officer for more than a year. Actually, there was little to be done other than routine maintenance, such as supervising the repair of the road "from the deposit of wood to the garrison . . . the only passage for the garrison." As late as November 29, 1783, his signature appears on a return, and apparently he remained in the army until it was completely disbanded in December. All men were authorized five years' pay in lieu of half-pay for life, yet many of them never were paid. Years later David did receive a bounty land warrant for four hundred acres.

After his discharge David returned to Saybrook and, desperate for money, petitioned the Connecticut General Assembly for payment for his services to the state from April 23,

1777, to August 2, 1779. During this time, he said, he had devoted all his time and efforts to pursuing measures to destroy the enemy's shipping on the Connecticut coast. He had also spent a considerable sum of his own money. For all of this he had never received a penny. Now he asked for £79.8.6 for expenses, and £410 in wages, at the rate of £15 a month. It was a modest request.

The petition was referred to a committee, and the committee debated and debated and debated. The state treasury already had been drained; there was no money to toss about freely. And Jonathan Trumbull no longer was Governor. Finally the committee reached a decision. No stated reward had been offered, it said, nor had David specifically been engaged to serve the state for the period he claimed. Also, the committee added, any reward "ought to depend in Some measure on the Success of his Views." Instead of the £489.8.6 he requested, he was granted £150, scarcely much capital with which to begin life all over again.

Misfortune continued to plague him. In 1785 he was stricken with a severe illness—exactly what is not known—which incapacitated him for nearly two years. And in February, 1786, his greatest friend and comrade—his brother Ezra—died.

Just about the time David became ill, a French inventor contrived a method of moving a vessel underwater by means of a screw propeller. It came to the attention of Thomas Jefferson, Minister Plenipotentiary to France from the United States. Recalling the *Turtle*, Jefferson suspected that perhaps David Bushnell deserved credit for having first discovered the use of the screw.

Actually, David never claimed credit for this discovery, and the use of a screw propeller had been discussed by others —notably Robert Hooke—before him. However, to obtain more information about the *Turtle*, Jefferson sent off letters to several friends, including Ezra Stiles and George Washington.

Washington replied in a letter from Mount Vernon dated September 26, 1785. "I am sorry that I cannot give you full information respecting Bushnell's projects for the destruction of ships," he said. "Bushnell is a man of great mechanical powers, fertile in inventions and master of execution . . . I then thought, and still think, that it was an effort of genius, but that too many things were necessary to be combined, to expect much from the issue against an enemy, who were always on guard." Davie Humphreys, Washington suggested, might be able to furnish a fuller account.

Both Humphreys and Stiles told David Bushnell of Jefferson's interest, yet not until October, 1787, had he recovered sufficiently from his illness to be able to write to Jefferson.

"I have ever carefully concealed my principles and experiments," he wrote, "as much as the nature of the subject allowed, from all but my chosen friends, being persuaded that it was the most prudent course, whether the event should prove fortunate or otherwise, although by the concealment, I never fostered any great expectations of profit, or even of a compensation for my time and expenses, the loss of which has been exceedingly detrimental to me."

With his letter, David sent Jefferson a full description of the *Turtle* and his experiments with her and with his mines. This description, it seems, may have been written years earlier, back in 1778, and submitted as one of the requirements for his Master's degree at Yale.

David forwarded the original of his letter to Jefferson in the care of Davie Humphreys, and, always cautious, he sent a copy of it to Ezra Stiles in case the original miscarried. To Stiles he wrote, "I could wish that what I have written should not come to the knowledge of the public, for the same reason, as I have written to the Governor, that I have ever wished to be silent upon the subject." He added that he could be reached, if necessary, in care of Major John Davenport in Stamford, who had been a tutor when he was a student at Yale.

Thirteen years after David sent his account of the *Turtle* to Jefferson a new submarine was tested in the Seine at Paris. This was the *Nautilus,* invented by the bumptious Robert Fulton.

There was a tone of more than slight contempt in the way Fulton dismissed David Bushnell's contributions. "In what Mr. Bushnal did there was much ingenuity," he wrote, "and no one respects his talents more than I do; had he prosecuted his studies, he probably might have perfected thought after thought to the annihilation of all ships of war. But whether his mind only viewed the subject as limited to little operations, or whether he thought too many difficulties attended it, he certainly did not compose his machines so as to make them of any use, nor did he organize anything like a system; and perhaps it is for these reasons that he had abandoned the subject for more than twenty-five years, and it is now dormant in him."

Fulton carefully neglected to mention what was undoubtedly his own debt to the inventions of David Bushnell. As a young man, Fulton had been a protegé of Benjamin Franklin, and Franklin had an intimate knowledge of the *Turtle* and how she worked. By the time Fulton built the *Nautilus,* he had been living for three years in the home of Joel Barlow and Barlow's wife, who was Abraham Baldwin's sister. Both Barlow and Baldwin had been friends of David Bushnell, and both had been in the Continental Army around New York at the time the *Turtle* attacked the *Eagle.* Moreover, in 1798, two years before Fulton began building the *Nautilus,* Bushnell's description sent to Jefferson had been read to the members of the American Philosophical Society and in 1799 the description had been published in the Society's *Transactions*.

And an examination of Fulton's diagrams for the *Nautilus* reveal many similarities to the *Turtle*. Fulton used a conning tower much like David's. He allowed space in the keel to hold water when the submarine submerged, as David had done. His screw propeller was an improvement over the one David had used, but it was modeled upon it. And his device for attaching a torpedo to a ship's hull and the torpedo itself were almost identical with David's.

Contemporaries were quick to point out that Fulton may have improved upon what David Bushnell did, but that his debt was great. In 1808, a writer in the English *Naval Chronicle*, after noting that Fulton often used the alias "Francis," went on to say, "The invention is at least ten years old, and is attributed to a Mr. Bushnell; so that unless Mr. F. can make out a right to that name by an additional *alias*, he is liable to the imputation of having received our money under false pretenses." (The English had paid Fulton liberally for some experiments he made.)

In 1813 Thomas Jefferson also came to David's defense, criticizing a recent naval history of the United States that had slighted the inventor. Writing to a friend, he said that the *Turtle* "was excellently contrived, and might perhaps, by improvement, be brought into real use. . . . It would be to the United States the consummation of their safety."

But David Bushnell's own voice was never heard in his defense. Indeed, so far as his family and friends in Connecticut were aware, he had disappeared not long after writing to Jefferson in 1787. On December 14, 1787, he had communicated with Captain Thomas Machin in New York about conveying the right David held to six hundred acres of land

between Seneca and Cayuga Lakes to his friend John Davenport. The right, David wrote, had been bought by him for
£30.6.0, and he had sold it to Major Davenport for a considerable sum.

About this time he had been staying with Ezra's family.
One day he announced that he had received letters from France
suggesting that he journey there to pursue his experiments on
the submarine and underwater mines. He could not make
up his mind whether or not to go, he said, but if he did decide
to risk the trip, he would send for his trunk.

Then he left the house. A few days later a note arrived
directing that the trunk be sent to New London. And at that
point he seemed to disappear.

All sorts of rumors circulated as to what had become of
him. It was said that he had actually gone to France, and that
he had perished in the French Revolution. It was said that he
had returned from abroad with a fortune, invested it in a
stock company in New Jersey, lost every penny, and disappeared once more.

But no one really knew.

XIV ➤ A Grave and Mysterious Man

SOMETIME IN the late 1780's a grave and mysterious man appeared at the Georgia home of Abraham Baldwin, Class of '72 at Yale, who had moved to Georgia early in 1784 and become active in politics.

The stranger was apparently ten or fifteen years older than Baldwin, strangely reticent about his past, and he did not put himself out to be friendly. Who this man of mystery was, and where he came from, no one knew, and Abraham Baldwin did not tell them. He simply introduced his friend as David Bush.

It soon was evident to those in this frontier state that David Bush was a man of considerable intelligence and unusual learning. And if he chose to keep to himself, that was none of their business. With Baldwin's help, it is said, he obtained a good position as a teacher, and old records indicate that he was among the original settlers of Columbia County, Georgia, created late in 1790. His ways were quiet, attracting little attention, and he left behind few traces:

On December 6, 1803, Jeremiah and Elizabeth Beall, for fifty dollars, sold David Bush a lot forty by eighty feet, lying south of the courthouse in Warrenton, Warren County, Georgia.

In 1810, when Warrenton was incorporated as a town, David Bush was one of the commissioners; in 1818 his name appeared as a practicing physician.

On June 8, 1820, in Augusta, David Bush made his will. It contained a stipulation which must have aroused the curiosity of anyone who read it:

"I give and bequeath unto George Hargraves, Esquire, of the City of Augusta, and Peter Crawford of the County of Columbia and State aforesaid, all my goods, and chattles, Lands and Tenements, and property of every description, that I may be in possession of or entitled to, at the time of my death: In Trust, to and for, the sole use and benefit of such person or persons; or for such uses and purposes as I may in a confidential manner, direct by written instructions under my hand and seal."

In the 1820 census for Habersham County, Georgia, the name of David Bush appears, his household consisting of one slave; and on June 21, 1824, he loaned $540 to William Hutchinson and James Culbreath, receiving a mortgage on 500 acres of land on Little River in Columbia County. Before the next year was out, he had loaned $9,006,06 to others, most of it to his friend George Hargraves. For all his eccentric secrecy, his guarded manner of speaking, his distant and forbidding attitude, he was considered a remarkable man, prosperous, thrifty, and still sharp-witted, though obviously well past eighty.

Then, sometime in January or early February, 1826, Dr. David Bush died. His will was probated in Augusta on February 6, and by May the inventory and appraisal of his estate had been completed. In addition to the notes for $9,546.06, it consisted, according to the court records, of "One Sorrel Horse" and "One old Gig and Harness," worth $125.

An astounding revelation was contained in the confidential

instructions to George Hargraves: the mysterious Dr. David Bush of Georgia, and David Bushnell, inventor of the *Turtle*, were the same person.

The estate was to go to Franklin College of the University of Georgia, founded by Abraham Baldwin, unless blood relations could be discovered in Saybrook who had "fair claims on the score of moral worth to such bounty." Heirs were discovered among Ezra Bushnell's children.

According to several reports, the estate contained one item not listed in the court inventory: "some curious machinery, partly built, which had been viewed by several gentlemen, none of whom had been able to determine what it would have been had it been completed." It is said that this was an uncompleted model for a new submarine torpedo, about which Dr. Bush had written to the Secretary of the Navy shortly before his death. If so, the secret of its workings died with him.

David Bushnell probably never traveled to France and obviously did not perish during the French Revolution. No doubt he went straight from Connecticut to Georgia. But where he studied medicine, why he never sent word of his whereabouts to his mother and friends in Connecticut, and why he concealed his identity for nearly half his life, is a mystery which, to this day, has never been solved.

XV ➤ The Father of
Submarine Warfare

DAVID BUSHNELL did everything he could to keep his name from being remembered. He cloaked his actions in secrecy. He never married, he cut himself off from his family, he made few close friends, and for the last forty years of his life he lived under an assumed name. He wrote few letters in an era when letter writing was a national pastime, and when he did write, he begged his correspondents not to divulge the contents of his letters.

He was helped on his way to obscurity by Robert Fulton, one of the world's most energetic press agents, who had no scruples about claiming David Bushnell's ideas as his own. Fulton's submarine, the *Nautilus*, had no greater practical success than the *Turtle*, and although the notion of anchoring mines was original with Fulton, his attempts at mine warfare were less successful than Bushnell's.

Yet before his death in 1815 Fulton had designed and built the *Clermont*, and his name is remembered, his achievements praised.

David Bushnell, who lived on until 1826, hid from fame behind the role of a country doctor. He hid well. Today few people have heard his name, and even fewer have any idea of how remarkable his achievements really were.

He invented the first practical submarine of which we have any reliable record. It fulfilled all the basic requirements: it was submersible, maneuverable, and it carried an adequate air supply.

He was the first man to conceive of a submarine as an offensive weapon in warfare.

He was the originator of mine warfare.

He did all this despite poor health, lack of money, and a passionate aversion to publicity and the advantages it might have. And he labored in a war waged by ragged, starving men who had little energy and less opportunity to support a genuinely new and unorthodox mode of attacking the enemy.

David Bushnell has remained a comparatively obscure genius even though the *Turtle* was fully as amazing a feat for the eighteenth century as the spaceship is for the twentieth century. Yet, almost in spite of himself, Bushnell has not gone entirely without his due.

Thomas Edison termed him "The Father of Submarine Warfare."

The United States Navy has named two submarine tenders in his honor, one in 1915 and another in 1942. The second USS *Bushnell*, nicknamed the "Turtle," played an important role during World War II in support of the submarines that struck paralyzing blows at Japanese sea power.

And, just recently, Congress passed a resolution urging the Navy to place David Bushnell's name upon a Polaris submarine. "It would be fitting," stated the resolution, "that such a vessel bear the name of the man who for the first time incorporated all the basic devices that make the modern submarine practical."

Words echo back from the past . . . Washington writing that "it was an effort of genius" . . . "Old Put" stating "It is possible that he may be considered of less consequence than he actually is" . . . and the Connecticut delegates to Congress, nearly two centuries ago, saying, "We are fully of the opinion that his genious ought to be encouraged and Rewarded."

Perhaps, in time, it may be.

Notes

(With a few exceptions, these notes refer only to material dealing directly with David Bushnell, his submarine, and his mines. Abbreviated citations refer to items listed fully in the Bibliography that follows.)

The quotation from Jefferson opposite the first page of the text is from Julian P. Boyd (ed.), *The Papers of Thomas Jefferson*, VIII, 300. The quotation from Washington is from Jared Sparks (ed.), *The Writings of Washington*, IX, 134-35.

CHAPTER I

The letter from Samuel Osgood to John Adams appears in Allen, *A Naval History of the American Revolution*, I, 153.

CHAPTER II

For facts about the life of David Bushnell and his family I have drawn mainly upon *American Biographical Dictionary*, 174; *Bushnell Family Genealogy*, Entries 160, 366-369; Field, *Stat. Account*, 97, 105, 138; Hinman, *Puritan Settlers*, 447; Howe, *American Mechanics*, 136; *Vital Records of Saybrook*, 140.

Based on the details available, I have reconstructed certain thoughts of David Bushnell and his father, which I believe to be accurate in all essentials. Although it has been said that Sarah Ingham was Nehemiah Bushnell's second wife, I could unearth no evidence to support this statement.

CHAPTERS III–IV

The description of David traveling to Yale by stage is my reconstruction of what most likely happened.

Notes

The two major sources for details about David Bushnell's experiments and the building of the *Turtle* are his description published in the *Transactions of the American Philosophical Society* and the letter from Benjamin Gale to Benjamin Franklin, August 7, 1775, in the manuscripts of the *Franklin Papers*, IV, Part 1, No. 61, American Philosophical Society. The account in the *Transactions* was originally enclosed with a letter from Bushnell to Thomas Jefferson, October, 1787. The originals of the description and the letter are in the New Haven Colony Historical Society's manuscript collections. The letter from Gale to Franklin is the earliest of his letters about the *Turtle* that has come to light. In this letter Gale mentions that the submarine has been completed except for the mine and that several tests have been made by David himself. As this letter is dated only twelve days after Bushnell's graduation from Yale, it leads me to conclude that construction of the *Turtle* must have begun during the period classes at Yale were suspended after news of Lexington and Concord.

The exact site where Bushnell built the *Turtle* is not stated in any contemporary records; tradition says it was either on Sill's Point or on Poverty Island, and evidence points more strongly toward Poverty Island.

Timothy Dwight, a tutor part of the time David was a student at Yale, later eulogized him in *Greenfield Hill* (VII, 431–4):

> See Bushnell's strong, creative genius, fraught
> With all th' assembled powers of skilful thought,
> His mystic vessel plunge beneath the waves,
> And glide thro' dark retreats, and coral caves!

CHAPTER V

In this chapter, too, I have used Bushnell's letter to Jefferson and Gale's letter to Franklin, both mentioned earlier. I have also drawn upon the following letters from Benjamin Gale to Silas Deane which appear in Conn. Hist. Soc., *Coll.*, II: November 9, 1775 (315–17); November 22, 1775 (322–23); December 7, 1775 (333–34); February 1, 1776 (358–59).

Here and later I have drawn upon the letter from Ezra Lee to David Humphreys published in *Mag. Am. Hist.*, March, 1893.

The quotation from the August 7, 1775, letter from Gale to Franklin appears at the bottom of the second page and top of the third page in the manuscript in the *Franklin Papers*, cited before. The letter from John Lewis is in *Lit. Diary Ezra Stiles*, I, 600.

The early report from a spy in the American camp which may refer to the *Turtle* is in "Spy's Letter," September 24, 1775, in the *Gage Papers*, William L. Clements Library.

The intelligence report from Tryon to Shuldham appears in *The Despatches of Molyneux Shuldham*, 41. A portion of it appears in *Hist. Maritime Conn.*, I, 160–1. The original is in the Public Record Office, London (Admiralty I/484). Details of Bushnell's appearances before the Council of Safety are recorded in Hinman's *Conn. during the War of the Rev.*, 343; in *Public Records Col. Conn.*, XV, 233–35; and in Connecticut State Library, Connecticut Archives Manuscripts, Revolutionary War 1763–1789, Series 2, Volume IV, 2b.

CHAPTERS VI–VIII

Most of the details about the exploits of the *Turtle* are taken from the description sent by Bushnell to Jefferson and from Lee's letter to Humphreys. The tradition (erroneous, I believe) that Washington viewed the *Turtle* when passing through Saybrook in April, 1776, appears in *Saybrook Colony 1635–1935*, among other places. William Williams' letter to Joseph Trumbull was published in *Letters of Members of the Continental Congress*, II, 42.

The comments of Washington about Bushnell quoted in this chapter and elsewhere are taken from his letter to Thomas Jefferson, September 26, 1785, published in Sparks' edition of *The Writings of Washington*, IX, 134–35. (It also appears in Ford's edition, X, 504, and in Fitzgerald's edition, XXVIII, 280–81.)

In Chapter VII, the letter from Parsons to Heath appears in Hall, *Parsons*, 60. Humphreys' statement about the *Turtle* is in Humphreys, *Putnam*, 108–112. In Chapter VIII, the remark by Heath is from *Heath*, 69.

CHAPTER IX

In this chapter the details about Bushnell's mines and about the attack on the *Cerberus* are drawn from Bushnell's letter to Jefferson, October, 1787, and from the official report of Commodore John Symons to Rear Admiral Sir Peter Parker, August 15, 1777. Details about Bushnell's appearance before the Council of Safety are recorded in Hinman's *Conn. during the War of the Rev.*, 437, and in *Public Records State of Conn.*, I, 212.

Notes

The letter from Parsons to Trumbull, November 2, 1777, is found in Mass. Hist. Soc. *Coll.*, 7th Ser., II (The Trumbull Papers, Part III), 183. The letter from Hopkinson (and John Wharton) to Washington is filed under its date, 17 December 1777, in Vol. 63 (leaves 7548A–B), *Washington Papers*, Manuscript Division, The Library of Congress. It also appears in Hastings, *Life and Works of Hopkinson*, 290–91.

Details about the Battle of the Kegs are drawn from Bushnell's letter to Jefferson, October, 1787, and from the letter, probably written by Hopkinson, published in the *New Jersey Gazette*, January 21, 1778, page 3, and in the *Continental Journal and Weekly Advertiser*, February 19, 1778, page 3. Hopkinson's ballad, "British Valour Displayed: Or, The Battle of the Kegs," first appeared in the *Pennsylvania Packet*, March 4, 1778, page 4. Among other papers in which it appeared was the *Continental Journal and Weekly Advertiser*, March 26, 1778, page 4. A copy in Hopkinson's writing is in the *Franklin Papers*, LXI, 1, No. 95, American Philosophical Society. A Tory rebuttal to Hopkinson's account of the Battle of the Kegs appeared in the *Pennsylvania Ledger*, February 11, 1778, and is published in Moore, *Diary of the Am. Rev.*, II, 7. For information about the Bordentown participants in what was known locally as "The Mechanical Kegs Plot," I have relied mainly upon the account in Woodward and Hageman, *Hist. of Burlington and Mercer Counties*, I, 463.

Reports on the damage done by the floating mines in the Battle of the Kegs are confused, and the destruction of the rowboat and the barge may, in fact, have been only one incident, not two separate ones.

On July 15, 1791, Claypoole's *American Daily Advertiser* noted that among the acquisitions of Peale's Museum in Philadelphia was ". . . a keg intended to have been used with those that were employed in the Delaware in the late war, as humourously discribed by Mr. Francis Hopkinson in *The Song of the Battle of the Kegs*." The museum's collections were dispersed long ago, and it is not known what became of the keg.

As first published in the *Pennsylvania Packet*, "British Valour Displayed: Or, The Battle of the Kegs" began:

> Gallants attend, and hear a friend
> Trill forth harmonious ditty;
> Strange things I'll tell, which late befel
> In Philadelphia city.

'Twas early day, as Poets say,
  Just when the sun was rising;
A soldier stood on a log of wood
  And saw a sight surprising.

As in a maze he stood to gaze,
  The truth can't be deny'd, Sir;
He spy'd a score of kegs, or more,
  Come floating down the tide, Sir

The complete ballad may be found in any number of collections of poetry.

CHAPTER XI

Bushnell's appearance before the Council of Safety in April, 1778, is recorded in Hinman's *Conn. during the War of the Rev.*, 531, and in *Public Records State of Conn.*, I, 580. The letter of the Connecticut delegates to Trumbull appears in Burnett, *Letters of Members of the Continental Congress*, III, 202. The statements by Ezra Stiles about the Master's candidates is from *Lit. Diary Ezra Stiles*, II, 301. The letter from Parsons to Trumbull has been published in Mass. Hist. Soc. Coll., 7th Ser., II (The Trumbull Papers, Part III), 374. The letter from Putnam to Washington about Bushnell's capture is from Sparks, *Corres. Am. Rev.*, II, 294–95.

The story of David's playing the fool aboard the prison ship appears in *History of Middlesex County*, 577. Details about the exchange of prisoners are recorded in *Public Records State of Conn.*, II, 289–90, and in Connecticut State Library, Connecticut Archives Manuscripts, Revolutionary War 1763–1789, Series 2, Vol. XIV, 381–383a. The letter of recommendation from Trumbull to Washington, May 29, 1779, appears in Stuart, *Life of Trumbull*, 294–95.

CHAPTERS XII–XIII

Information about David Bushnell's service in the Corps of Sappers and Miners may be found in *Record of Service of Conn. Men*, 298; Heitman's *Historical Register*, 110; and in Fitzpatrick (ed.), *Writings of Washington*, XVI, 35–36, 121; XVII, 443–44; XXII, 234, 411; XXVI, 129–31, 168; XXVII, 154. Additional details are found in the service record for David Bushnell compiled by the National Archives and in National Archives Microfilms Publications, Microcopy No. 246,

Notes

Revolutionary War Rolls 1775–1783, Roll 122, Continental Troops, Jacket Number 77, 1–14.

Information about his petitions to the Connecticut General Assembly during the period covered by this chapter may be found in *Public Records State of Conn.*, III, 160; IV, 194; V, 395; and in Connecticut State Library, Connecticut Archives Manuscripts, Revolutionary War 1763–1789, Series 2, XVII, 328; XXI, 69b; XXII, 369–70; XXVII, 115–18; XXVIII, 197; and in Revolutionary War June 1765—May 1782, I, 12a.

The quotation from the orders directing the Sappers and Miners to march at the head of the column is taken from Fitzpatrick (ed.), *Writings of Washington*, XVI, 48. Further details about David Bushnell's career in the Sappers and Miners are found in Martin (Scheer, ed.), *Private Yankee Doodle*, 195–280; however, contrary to the editor's note, the "captain" referred to by Martin was not always David Bushnell.

In Chapter XIII, the dialogue of Taulman and Kirkpatrick is quoted directly from a letter from Captain David Bushnell to Major General Henry Knox, January 2, 1783, in the Massachusetts Historical Society. Washington's comments after the court-martial are found in Fitzpatrick (ed.), *Writings of Washington*, XXVI, 131.

The order directing Captain Bushnell to repair the road to the garrison appears in Johnston, *Yale in the Rev.*, 308. The records of the Veterans Administration in the National Archives contain the notation that Bounty Land Warrant No. 141 for 300 acres of land was issued on February 3, 1800, based on the service of Captain David Bushnell of the Corps of Sappers and Miners; no papers are on file relating to this warrant.

When the Society of the Cincinnati was formed in June, 1783, by officers of the Continental Army for the purpose of preserving the bonds of their friendship, Captain David Bushnell became one of the members.

The various publications in which Washington's letter to Jefferson, September 26, 1785, may be found have been cited in the notes for Chapters VI–VIII. Thomas Jefferson's letters to Ezra Stiles and George Washington about Bushnell may be found in Boyd (ed.), *The Papers of Thomas Jefferson*, VIII, 299–300; an earlier letter about "the Connecticut turtle," to Hugh Williamson is in VII, 642–43. David Bushnell's reply to Jefferson, October, 1787 (with which he enclosed the description of his inventions and experiments) has been published in Boyd (ed.), *The Papers of Thomas Jefferson*, XII, 303–304. The original of this letter is in the New Haven Colony Historical Society, as is Bushnell's letter to Ezra Stiles in which he reiterates his desire for secrecy.

Fulton's attack on Bushnell appears in his *Letters Principally to the Right Honourable Lord Grenville*, 32–33. The quotation from the *Naval Chronicle* appears in XX, 452.

Jefferson's defense of Bushnell appears in Lipscomb (ed.), *The Writings of Thomas Jefferson*, XIII, 263.

The letter from David Bushnell to Captain Thomas Machin, December 14, 1787, is in the Stokes Manuscripts, Yale University Library. The information about David Bushnell's intention to leave for France is found in a letter from James H. Manning to Anson Phelps Stokes, November 7, 1912, in the Stokes Manuscripts, Yale University Library; Manning quotes a statement made by Ezra Bushnell, David's nephew, in 1826.

CHAPTER XIV

Reasonably accurate information about David Bushnell's life in Georgia is recorded in Sherwood, *Gazetteer*, 250; Knight, *Georgia's Landmarks*, I, 480–81, 1015–16; II, 1019; and in White, *Historical Coll. of Georgia*, 406, 409. The deed to Bushnell from Jeremiah and Elizabeth Beall is in *Georgia, Warren Co. Superior Court Deed Book B, 1801–1808*, 455–56.

A manuscript volume *Executive Department, Georgia, Louisville, 19th July 1805* shows that Doctor David Bush was entitled to one draw in Georgia's First Land Lottery, also known as the 1805 Lottery, and that he drew a blank, therefore gaining no land as a bounty.

The copy of David Bushnell's will is in *Richmond County Ordinary's Office–Estate Records–Wills, 1798–1853*, Vol. 8, SLC 255–256, 249–50. The mortgage from Hutchinson and Culbreath is in *Columbia County, Georgia, Deeds and Mortgages Book X, 1822–1824*, 468–69. Record of the probate of the will is in *Richmond County–Augusta, Ga. Estate Records Book 2-B*, 54. The inventory and appraisal of his estate is in *Richmond County, Georgia Inventories . . . Suppt. Book C, 1823–1829*, 302. The last six items are either on file or on microfilm in the Georgia Department of Archives and History.

CHAPTER XV

The quotation by Edison is from *In the Land of the Patentees*. The resolution of the House and Senate is quoted as it appeared in the *New London Day*, April 19, 1961.

Bibliography

I. PRIMARY MATERIAL ON THE LIFE, INVENTIONS AND EXPLOITS OF DAVID BUSHNELL

BOOKS AND PUBLISHED COLLECTIONS

Abbot, Henry L., Compiler. *The Beginning of Modern Submarine Warfare under Captain-Lieutenant David Bushnell, Sappers and Miners, Army of the Revolution.* Willets Point, New York Harbor: The Battalion press, 1881.

Allen, Gardner W. *A Naval History of the American Revolution.* 2 vols. Boston: Houghton Mifflin Company, 1913.

Burnett, Edmund C., Editor. *Letters of Members of the Continental Congress.* 8 vols. Washington, D.C.: Carnegie Institution of Washington, 1921–1936.

Bushnell, George Eleazer. *Bushnell Family Genealogy.* Nashville, Tenn.: Privately printed, 1945.

Connecticut. *The Public Records of the Colony of Connecticut.* 15 vols. Hartford: Case, Lockwood & Brainard Company, 1850–1890.

———. *The Public Records of the State of Connecticut.* Vol. I- . Hartford: Case, Lockwood & Brainard Company, 1894-   .

———. *Record of Service of Connecticut Men in the War of the Revolution.* Compiled by Authority of the General Assembly, Under Direction of the Adjutants General. Hartford: Case, Lockwood & Brainard Company, 1889.

Connecticut Historical Society. *Collections.* Vol. II (Correspondence of Silas Deane, Delegate to the First and Second Congress at Philadelphia). Hartford: Published for the Society, 1870.

———. *Collections.* Vol. XX (Huntington Papers). Hartford: Published for the Society, 1923.

Field, David D. *A Statistical Account of the County of Middlesex in Connecticut.* Middletown, Conn.: Connecticut Academy of Arts and Sciences, 1819.

Fulton, Robert. *Letters Principally to the Right Honourable Lord Grenville on Sub-Marine Navigation and Attack.* . . . London: S. Gosnell, 1806.

Hall, Charles S. *Life and Letters of Samuel Holden Parsons.* Binghamton, N.Y.: Otseningo Publishing Company, 1905.

Hastings, George Everett. *The Life and Works of Francis Hopkinson.* Chicago: The University of Chicago Press, 1926.

Heath, William. *Memoirs of Major-General William Heath.* Edited by William Abbatt. New York: W. Abbatt, 1901.

Heitman, Francis B. *Historical Register of Officers of the Continental Army during the War of the Revolution, April, 1775, to December, 1783.* Washington, D.C.: W. H. Lowdermilk & Company, 1893.

Hinman, Royal. *A Catalog of the Names of the Early Puritan Settlers of the Colony of Connecticut.* Hartford: Case, Tiffany and Company, 1852.

————. *A Historical Collection, From Official Records, Files, &c., of the Part Sustained by Connecticut during the War of the Revolution.* Hartford: E. Gleason, 1842.

Humphreys, David. *An Essay on the Life of the Honourable Major General Israel Putnam.* Boston: Samuel Avery, 1818.

Jefferson, Thomas. *The Papers of Thomas Jefferson.* Edited by Julian P. Boyd, *et al.* Vol. I– . Princeton: Princeton University Press, 1950– .

————. *The Writings of Thomas Jefferson.* Monticello Edition. Andrew A. Lipscomb, Editor-in-Chief. 20 vols. Washington, D.C.: The Thomas Jefferson Memorial Association, 1904–5.

Martin, Joseph Plumb. *Private Yankee Doodle, Being a Narrative of Some of the Adventures, Dangers and Sufferings of a Revolutionary Soldier.* Edited by George F. Scheer. Boston: Little, Brown and Company, 1962.

Massachusetts Historical Society. *Collections.* 7th Series. Vol. II (The Trumbull Papers. Part III). Boston: Published by the Society, 1902.

Middlebrook, Louis F. *History of Maritime Connecticut During the American Revolution 1775–1783.* 2 vols. Salem, Mass.: The Essex Institute, 1925.

Moore, Frank. *Diary of the American Revolution.* 2 vols. New York: Charles Scribner, 1860.

Shuldham, Molyneux. *The Despatches of Molyneux Shuldham, Vice-Admiral of the Blue and Commander-in-Chief of His Britannic Majesty's Ships in North America January–July 1776.* Edited by Robert Wilden Neeser. New York: Printed for the Naval History Society by the De Vinne Press, 1913.

Sparks, Jared, Editor. *Correspondence of the American Revolution.* 4 vols. Boston: Little, Brown, and Company, 1853.

Stiles, Ezra. *The Literary Diary of Ezra Stiles, D.D., LL.D.* Edited by Franklin Bowditch Dexter. 3 vols. New York: Charles Scribner's Sons, 1901.

Stuart, I. W. *Life of Jonathan Trumbull, Sen., Governor of Connecticut.* Boston: Crocker and Brewster, 1859.

Vital Records of Saybrook 1647–1834. Hartford: The Connecticut Historical Society and the Connecticut Society of the Order of the Founders and Patriots of America, 1852.

Washington, George. *The Writings of George Washington.* Edited by John C. Fitzpatrick. 39 vols. Washington, D.C.: Government Printing Office, 1931–1944.

———. *The Writings of George Washington.* Edited by Worthington Chauncey Ford. 14 vols. New York: G. P. Putnam's Sons, 1889–1893.

———. *The Writings of George Washington.* Edited by Jared Sparks. 12 vols. New York: Harper & Brothers, 1847–1848.

PERIODICALS

Bushnell, David. "General Principles and Construction of a Submarine Vessel." *Transactions of the American Philosophical Society,* Vol. IV (1799), No. 37, 303–312.

Claypoole's *American Daily Advertiser,* July 15, 1791.

Continental Journal and Weekly Advertiser (Boston), February 19, 1778; March 26, 1778.

Lee, Ezra. "Letter from Ezra Lee to General David Humphreys, Lyme, 20th February 1815." *Magazine of American History,* March, 1893.

New Jersey Gazette (Burlington), January 21, 1778.

Pennsylvania Ledger (Philadelphia), February 11, 1778.

Pennsylvania Packet (Lancaster), March 4, 1778.

The Remembrancer or Impartial Repository of Public Events for the Year 1778 (Report of Commodore John Symons to Admiral Sir Peter Parker), VI, 90–91.

MANUSCRIPTS

David Bushnell Letter to Henry Knox, Massachusetts Historical Society.

David Bushnell Letters to Ezra Stiles and Thomas Jefferson, New Haven Colony Historical Society.

Connecticut Archives, Revolutionary War, Connecticut State Library.

Franklin Papers, American Philosophical Society.

Gage Papers, William L. Clements Library, University of Michigan.

Georgia Archives, Records of Columbia, Habersham, Richmond and Warren Counties, Georgia Department of Archives and History.

Revolutionary War Rolls, National Archives.

Anson Phelps Stokes Manuscripts, Yale University Library.

U.S. Army Miscellaneous Papers, New York Public Library.

II. SECONDARY MATERIAL ON DAVID BUSHNELL, THE *TURTLE* AND THE BATTLE OF THE KEGS

(NOTE: This list is highly selective and omits the numerous brief —and usually inaccurate—accounts of Bushnell and the *Turtle*.)

BOOKS

Abbott, Katharine M. *Old Paths and Legends of the New England Border.* New York: G. P. Putnam's Sons, 1907.

Allen, William. *The American Biographical Dictionary.* Third Edition. Boston: John P. Jewett and Company, 1857.

Appleton's Cyclopedia of American Biography. Edited by James Grant Wilson and John Fiske. New York: D. Appleton and Company, 1888.

Bakeless, John. *Turncoats, Traitors and Heroes.* Philadelphia: J. B. Lippincott and Company, 1959.

Barber, F. M. *Lecture on Submarine Boats and the Application to Torpedo Operations.* Newport, R.I.: U.S. Torpedo Station, 1875.

Barber, John W. *Connecticut Historical Collections.* New Haven: Durrie & Peck, 1836.

Barber, John W., and Howe, Henry. *Historical Collections of the*

State of New Jersey. New York: S. Tuttle, 1844.

Barnes, J. S. *Submarine Warfare, Offensive and Defensive.* New York: D. Van Nostrand, 1869.

Burgoyne, Alan H. *Submarine Navigation, Past and Present.* 2 vols. New York: E. P. Dutton & Company, 1903.

Caulkins, Frances Manwaring. *History of New London, Connecticut.* New York: H. D. Utley, 1895.

Crofut, Florence S. Marcy. *Guide to the History and the Historic Sites of Connecticut.* 2 vols. New Haven: Yale University Press, 1937.

Cutter, William. *The Life of Israel Putnam.* New York: Derby & Jackson, 1858.

Delpeuch, Maurice. *Les Sous-Marins a Travers Les Siècles.* Paris: Société d'Édition et de Publications, 1907.

Dexter, Franklin Bowditch. *Biographical Sketches of the Graduates of Yale College with Annals of the College History.* 6 vols. New York: Henry Holt and Company, 1885–1912.

Field, Cyril. *The Story of the Submarine.* Philadelphia: J. B. Lippincott Company, 1908.

Flexner, James Thomas. *Steamboats Come True: American Inventors in Action.* New York: The Viking Press, 1944.

Gates, Gilman C. *Saybrook at the Mouth of the Connecticut.* Orange, Conn.: Wilson H. Lee Company, 1935.

History of Middlesex County, Connecticut, with Biographical Sketches of Its Prominent Men. New York: J. B. Beers & Company, 1884.

History of Warren County, Georgia. Unpublished manuscript in the Georgia Department of Archives and History.

Hopkinson, Francis. *The Battle of the Kegs.* Illustrated Edition. Philadelphia: Oakwood Press, 1866.

Howe, Henry. *Memoirs of the Most Eminent American Mechanics.* New York: Derby & Jackson, 1858.

Humphreys, Francis L. *Life and Times of David Humphreys.* 2 vols. New York: G. P. Putnam's Sons, 1917.

In the Land of the Patentees: Saybrook in Connecticut. Second Edition Enlarged. Old Saybrook, Conn.: The Acton Library, 1935.

Johnston, Henry P. *Yale and Her Honor-Roll in the American Revolution 1775–1783.* New York: Privately printed, 1888.

Kingsley, William L. *Yale College: A Sketch of Its History.* 2 vols. New York: Henry Holt and Company, 1879.

Knight, Lucian Lamar. *Georgia's Landmarks, Memorials and*

Legends. 2 vols. Atlanta, Georgia: The Byrd Printing Company, 1913.

Magee, James D. *Bordentown 1682–1932.* Bordentown, N.J.: The Bordentown Register, 1932.

New Jersey: A Guide to Its Present and Past. Compiled and Written by the Federal Writers' Project of the Works Progress Administration of the State of New Jersey. New York: The Viking Press, 1939.

Parsons, Wm. Barclay. *Robert Fulton and the Submarine.* New York: Columbia University Press, 1922.

Pease, John C., and Niles, John M. *A Gazetteer of the States of Connecticut and Rhode-Island.* Hartford: William S. Marsh, 1819.

Pesce. G.-L. *La Navigation Sous-Marine.* Paris: Vuibert & Nony, 1906.

Scharf, J. Thomas, and Westcott, Thompson. *History of Philadelphia, 1609–1884.* 3 vols. Philadelphia: L. H. Everts Company, 1884.

Schieffelin, Edward Loomis. *David Bushnell and the First American Submarine.* Unpublished manuscript in the Connecticut State Library, the Submarine Library, and the Yale University Library.

Sherwood, Adiel. *A Gazetteer of the State of Georgia.* Third Edition. Washington, D.C.: P. Force, 1837.

Stokes, Anson Phelps. *Memorials of Eminent Yale Men.* 2 vols. New Haven: Yale University Press, 1914.

Thacher, James. *Military Journal of the American Revolution.* Hartford: Hurlbut, Williams & Company, 1862. (First published as *A Military Journal During the American Revolutionary War.* Boston, 1823.)

Tomlinson, E. *David Bushnell and His American Turtle.* New York: The Werner Company, 1899. (A fictionalized biography of Bushnell through the attack on the *Eagle.*)

Trumbull, Jonathan. *Jonathan Trumbull, Governor of Connecticut, 1769–1784.* Boston: Little, Brown and Company, 1919.

Tyler, Moses Coit. *The Literary History of the American Revolution 1763–1783.* 2 vols. New York and London: G. P. Putnam's Sons, 1897.

Watson, John F. *Annals of Philadelphia and Pennsylvania, in the Olden Times.* 2 vols. Philadelphia: Published by the author. 1844.

White, George. *Historical Collections of Georgia.* Third Edition. New York: Pudney & Russell, 1855.

Woodward, E. M., and Hageman, John F. *History of Burlington and Mercer Counties, New Jersey.* 2 vols. Philadelphia: Everts & Peck, 1883.

PERIODICALS AND PAMPHLETS

The American Journal of Science, 1820, 94.

Historic Pageant of Bordentown, New Jersey, Souvenir Program, 1917.

Historical Guide Published by the Bordentown Historical Society.

Magazine of American History, April, 1882, 297.

Naval Chronicle, XX, 452.

New London Day, April 19, 1961.

Sanders, Harry. "The First American Submarine." *United States Naval Institute Proceedings*, December, 1936, 1743–1745.

Saybrook Colony 1635–1935, Official Program of Tercentenary Celebration July 18–20, 1935.

Thomson, David W. "David Bushnell and the First American Submarine." *United States Naval Institute Proceedings*, February, 1942, 176–186.

III. BOOKS AND PERIODICALS ON THE REVOLUTION, ON YALE AND ON LIFE IN CONNECTICUT

(NOTE: These were the most helpful among the many books consulted to provide an authentic background for the story of David Bushnell.)

Adams, James Truslow. *Revolutionary New England 1691–1776.* Boston: Little, Brown, and Company, 1923.

Adams, John. *Diary and Autobiography of John Adams.* (Vols. 1–4 of The Adams Papers, L. H. Butterfield, Editor-in-Chief) Cambridge, Mass.: Harvard University Press, 1961.

Alden, John Richard. *The American Revolution.* New York: Harper & Brothers, 1954.

Anderson, Troyer S. *The Command of the Howe Brothers during the American Revolution.* New York and London: Oxford University Press, 1936.

Arnold, Isaac N. *The Life of Benedict Arnold.* Chicago: Jansen, McClurg & Company, 1880.

Baker, William S. *Itinerary of General Washington from June 15,*

1775, to December 23, 1783. Philadelphia: J. B. Lippincott Company, 1892.

Baldwin, Ebenezer. *Annals of Yale College.* Second Edition. New Haven: B. & W. Noyes, 1838.

Barrow, Sir John. *The Life of Richard, Earl Howe.* London: J. Murray, 1838.

Bliven, Bruce, Jr. *Battle for Manhattan.* New York: Henry Holt and Company, 1956.

Bowen, Catherine Drinker. *John Adams and the American Revolution.* Boston: Little, Brown and Company, 1950.

Boynton, E. C. *History of West Point.* New York: D. Van Nostrand, 1863.

Brooks, Noah. *Henry Knox.* New York: G. P. Putnam's Sons, 1900.

Calhoun, Arthur W. *A Social History of the American Family* (Vol. I: *The Colonial Period*). 3 vols. Cleveland: The Arthur H. Clark Company, 1917–1919.

Chapman, Edward M. *The First Church of Christ in Saybrook 1646–1946.* New Haven: Privately printed, 1947.

Chidsey, Donald Barr. *Valley Forge.* New York: Crown Publishers, Inc., 1959.

———. *Victory at Yorktown.* New York: Crown Publishers, Inc., 1962.

Chipman, Daniel. *The Life of Hon. Nathaniel Chipman, LL.D.* Boston: Charles C. Little and James Brown, 1846.

Clark, William Bell. *George Washington's Navy.* Baton Rouge, La.: Louisiana State University Press, 1960.

Cooper, J. Fenimore. *History of the Navy of the United States of America.* 2 vols. Cooperstown, N.Y.: H. & E. Phinney, 1848.

Davis, Matthew L. *Memoirs of Aaron Burr with Miscellaneous Selections from His Correspondence.* 2 vols. New York: Harper & Brothers, 1836–1837.

Decker, Malcolm. *Benedict Arnold.* Tarrytown, N.Y.: W. Abbatt, 1932.

Drake, Francis Samuel. *Life and Correspondence of Henry Knox.* Boston: S. G. Drake, 1873.

Durfee, Calvin. *Sketch of the Late Rev. Ebenezer Fitch, D.D., First President of Williams College.* Boston: Massachusetts Sabbath School Society, 1865.

Forbes, Esther. *Paul Revere & the World He Lived In.* Boston: Houghton Mifflin Company, 1942.

Ganoe, William Addleman. *The History of the United States Army.* Revised Edition. New York and London: D. Appleton-Century Company, 1943.

Bibliography

Gipson, Lawrence Henry. *The Coming of the Revolution*. New York: Harper & Brothers, 1954.

Hamilton, Alexander. *The Papers of Alexander Hamilton*. Harold C. Syrett, Editor. Vol. I– . New York: Columbia University Press, 1961– .

——. *The Works of Alexander Hamilton*. Edited by John C. Hamilton. 7 vols. New York: Charles S. Francis & Company, 1850–1851.

Howard, Leon. *The Connecticut Wits*. Chicago: The University of Chicago Press, 1943.

Hudleston, F. J. *Gentleman Johnny Burgoyne*. Indianapolis: The Bobbs-Merrill Company, 1927.

Irving, Washington. *The Life of Washington*. 3 vols. New York: Frank F. Lovell Company. 1856.

James, William M. *The British Navy in Adversity*. London and New York: Longmans, Green and Co. Ltd., 1926.

Johnston, Henry P. *The Yorktown Campaign and the Surrender of Cornwallis 1781*. New York: Harper & Brothers, 1881.

Kite, Elizabeth S. *Brigadier-General Louis Lebègue Duportail, Commandant of Engineers in the Continental Army, 1777–1783*. Baltimore: The Johns Hopkins Press, 1933.

Knox, Dudley W. *The Naval Genius of George Washington*. Boston: Houghton Mifflin Company, 1932.

Lancaster, Bruce. *From Lexington to Liberty*. Garden City, New York: Doubleday & Company, Inc., 1955.

Livingston, W. F. *Israel Putnam*. New York: G. P. Putnam's Sons, 1901.

Lossing, Benson J. *The Pictorial Field-Book of the Revolution*. 2 vols. New York: Harper & Brothers, 1855 and 1860.

Mahan, Alfred T. *The Major Operations of the Navies in the War of American Independence*. Boston: Little, Brown and Company, 1913.

Marcus, G. J. *A Naval History of England* (Vol. I: *The Formative Centuries*). Vol. I– . Boston: Little, Brown and Company, 1961– .

Morris, Richard B., Editor. *Encyclopedia of American History*. Revised and Enlarged Edition. New York: Harper & Brothers, 1961.

Parton, James. *Life and Times of Aaron Burr*. New York: Mason Bros., 1858.

——. *Life and Times of Benjamin Franklin*. 2 vols. New York: Mason Bros., 1865.

Paullin, Charles Oscar. *The Navy of the American Revolution.* Cleveland: Burrows Brothers, 1906.

Schachner, Nathan. *Aaron Burr.* New York: Frederick A. Stokes Company, 1937.

Scheer, George F., and Rankin, Hugh F. *Rebels and Redcoats.* Cleveland: The World Publishing Company, 1957.

Seymour, George Dudley. *Documentary Life of Nathan Hale.* New Haven: Privately printed, 1941.

Steiner, Bernard C. *The History of Education in Connecticut.* (Bureau of Education Circular of Information No. 2, 1893. Contributions to American Educational History, No. 14.) Washington, D.C.: Government Printing Office, 1893.

Van Dusen, Albert E. *Connecticut.* New York: Random House, 1961.

Wallace, Willard M. *Traitorous Hero: The Life and Fortunes of Benedict Arnold.* New York: Harper & Brothers, 1954.

Ward, Christopher. *The War of the Revolution.* Edited by John Richard Alden. 2 vols. New York: The Macmillan Company, 1952.

Warfel, Harry R. *Noah Webster, Schoolmaster to America.* New York: The Macmillan Company, 1936.

Weig, Melvin J. *Morristown: A Military Capital of the American Revolution.* (National Park Service Historical Handbook Series No. 7.) Washington, D.C.: Government Printing Office, 1950.

Woodward, Ashbel. *Memoir of Col. Thomas Knowlton of Ashford, Connecticut.* Boston: Henry W. Dutton & Son, 1861.

Zeichner, Oscar. *Connecticut's Years of Controversy 1750–1776.* Chapel Hill, N.C.: University of North Carolina Press, 1949.

Connecticut Gazette, May 31, 1766.

Connecticut Journal; and New-Haven Post-Boy, July 5, 1766; July 5, 1775; August 30, 1775.

New London Gazette, Nos. 152, 172.

Index

Index

Greene, Nathanael, 101
Griswold, Matthew, 38, 46

Habersham County, Georgia, 120
Hale, Nathan, 18, 20, 35, 68-70, 101
Halifax, Nova Scotia, 48, 49
Halley, Edmond, 17, 19
Hamilton, Alexander, 103, 106, 107
Hargraves, George, 120, 121
Harlem Heights, N.Y., 68
Hartford, Conn., 12, 94, 103
Harvard College, 15
Hayden, Uriah, 9
Head of Elk (Elkton), Md., 104
Heath, William, 58-59, 73
Hooke, Robert, 114
Hopkinson, Francis, 85-86, 88-89
Howe, Richard, 4th Viscount and 1st Earl Howe, 49, 50, 52, 58, 59, 64, 66, 79, 84, 88
Howe, Sir William, 5th Viscount Howe, 1, 47, 49, 52, 57, 68, 69, 79, 83, 84, 91
Hudson River, 48, 49, 50, 53, 59, 67, 68, 70-73, 83, 99-101, 104
Humphreys, David, 53, 59-60, 115
Hutchinson, William, 120

Ingersoll, Jared, 11-12

Jackaway, Robert, 85
Jefferson, Thomas, 52, 114-117

Kip's Bay, N.Y., 66, 67
Kirkpatrick, David, 106, 107, 111-112
Knox, Henry, 112
Knowlton, Thomas, 68

Lafayette, Marie Joseph Paul Yves Roch Gilbert du Motier, Marquis de, 96, 102, 106
Lebanon, Conn., 45, 77
Lee, Charles, 33
Lee, Ezra, 55, 59-65, 69-73
Lewis, John, 39
Lexington, Mass., 1, 2, 26, 27, 28, 30
Linonia Society, 20-21
Long Island, 57, 62, 69, 92-93
Long Island, battle of, 57-58, 64
Long Island Sound, 4, 8, 36-37, 55-56, 58
Loring, Joshua, 93-94

Lyme, Conn., 11, 23-24, 38, 48, 54, 55, 91

Machin, Thomas, 117-118
Manhattan Island, N.Y., 48, 57, 58-59, 62, 66-74
Middlesex, Conn., 92
mines, submarine, 22, 24-25, 39, 40-42, 60, 63-64, 76-77, 79-82, 83, 85-89, 94, 95, 118
Monmouth, battle of, 91
Morristown, N.J., 76, 98
Murray, Mrs. Robert, 68

Nautilus, 116-117, 122
New Haven, Conn., 3, 4, 7, 12, 14-15, 26-27, 31, 33, 39, 43, 48
New Jersey, 75, 99
New London, Conn., 48, 52, 79, 91, 118
New Rochelle, N.Y., 58
New York, N.Y., 9, 33, 47-50, 52, 66, 69, 83, 91, 98, 100, 103, 104, 109
New York Bay, 48, 58, 60-66, 79
Newport, R.I., 91
North River, N.Y., 58-59, 67

Osgood, Samuel, 3-4, 41

Parker, Sir Peter, 79, 81
Parliament, 10, 11, 23
Parsons, Samuel, 54-55, 58-59, 60, 66, 67, 83-84, 91-92, 94, 98
Peekskill, N.Y., 99, 101
Philadelphia, Pa., 4, 9, 32, 41, 49, 79, 83, 84, 86, 87, 89, 91, 101, 110
Phoenix, 49, 50, 53-54, 70, 72-73
Plowman, Joseph, 85
Pochaug, Conn., 5, 8, 9, 11, 75 (see also Saybrook)
Portsmouth, Va., 102
Poverty Island, Conn., 29, 35, 36
Putnam, Israel, 50-51, 53-54, 57, 59-60, 63, 66, 68, 76, 93-94, 123-124

Renown, 91
Rhode Island, 1, 3, 76, 79, 87
Roebuck, 70, 72-73, 88
Rose, 3, 49, 50, 53-54

Sappers and Miners, Corps of, 94, 96-99, 101-113

144

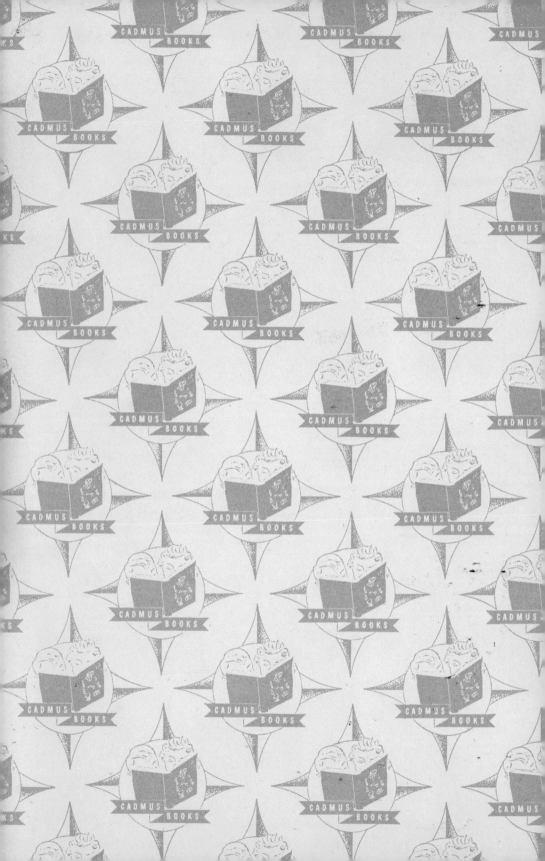